Waltzing with Jack Dancer

A Slow Dance with Cancer

Poems by Geoff Goodfellow
Story by Grace Goodfellow
Images by Randy Larcombe

16
EasyRead Large

RHYW

Copyright Page from the Original Book

Wakefield Press
1 The Parade West
Kent Town
South Australia 5067
www.wakefieldpress.com.au

First published 2011

Edited by Graham Rowlands
Story edited by Julia Beaven
Designed by Mark Thomas
Printing and quality control in China by Tingleman Pty Ltd

National Library of Australia Cataloguing-in-Publication entry

Author: Goodfellow, Geoff, 1949– .
Title: Waltzing with Jack Dancer: a slow dance with cancer / poems by Geoff Goodfellow; story by Grace Goodfellow; photographs by Randy Larcombe.
ISBN: 978 1 86254 959 3 (pbk.).
ISBN: 978 1 86254 961 6 (hbk.).
Subjects: Dancer, Jack.
Cancer – Patients – Australia – Biography.
Other Authors/Contributors: Goodfellow, Grace. Larcombe, Randy.
Dewey Number: 616.994092

Acknowledgements:
ABC 891 with Carole Whitelock
ABC Tasmania *Statewide Mornings* with Tim Cox
ABC TV *Stateline* with Leah MacLennan
A Million Bright Things CD
Best Australian Poetry 2009
Famous Reporter
Quit Anti-Smoking Campaign
Radio Adelaide *Arts Breakfast*
Radio Adelaide *Writers' Radio*
The Adelaide Review
The Advertiser: SA Weekend Magazine
The Record
The Weekend Australian
Wet Ink

A version of 'The C Word' was judged as the winning entry for the SA/NT division of the 2010 Somerset National Novella Award.

Government of South Australia
Arts SA

fox creek wines

Set in 16 pt. Verdana

TABLE OF CONTENTS

Also by Geoff Goodfellow

No Collars No Cuffs
Bow Tie & Tails
No Ticket No Start
Triggers: turning experiences into poetry
Triggers: the video
The Sex Poems Unleashed
Semi Madness: voices from Semaphore
Love is Cruel
Love is Cruel: spoken word+music CD
Poems for a Dead Father
Punch On Punch Off

For Guy Rees

Once you were in my corner
I knew I could go the distance.

Foreword

In January 2008 Geoff was admitted to the Queen Elizabeth Hospital with a sore throat. I took a number of messages and phone calls from him during that day. Generally they were angry calls but there was also a hint of anxiety as if he was already suspecting the worst. It was a very short SMS that finally communicated the diagnosis.

Throat cancer is one of several head and neck cancers. There is a strong link between head and neck cancers and the smoking of tobacco and cannabis and the drinking of alcohol. It is in many ways the baby boomers' disease. It is also in many ways the working man's disease and it was so described by Geoff's surgeon, Mr Guy Rees.

When I visited Geoff at home the first weekend after the diagnosis he was surrounded by friends and family. There was no doubt he had been dealt a massive blow. For the first time I saw him hunched over instead of leading with his chin. He was in a dressing gown and speaking softly. I thought he had met his match. I shouldn't have worried. He had not been beaten. Rather like a wily old boxer he'd simply taken some shelter on the ropes while he sized up his opponent.

By the time he had had his first meeting with 'The Seventh Doctor' the fight strategy had been well and truly set. The poem 'Another Fight' tells the story. Round by round Goodfellow came back.

On a wet winter's day I found my way to the bed in the public ward to which Geoff had been admitted only to find it empty. There was a moment of anxiety before I discovered that Geoff had, by fair means or foul managed to work his way into a private room overlooking the Botanic Gardens. The poem 'Night Moves' tells you how.

After many rounds it was ultimately a knock-out win. The cancer was vanquished and transformed by words into this important book. The use of the Australian rhyming slang for cancer to play on the image of the dancing boxer gives this work a strongly Australian theme.

The comparison between the gum-booted surgeon in 'The Seventh Doctor' and the imagery of a concrete finisher is stark. The real story here I think is that Geoff hoped that his surgeon was as skilled as the elite building tradesman he knew from his years on building sites. In 'Blue Sky Morning', yet another contrast between Australia's pristine blue skies and the tobacco saturated working lives of many blue-collar Australians in the post-war era. In 'Maybe' the glamour and machismo of cigarette advertising is contrasted with a cancer ward full of its victims.

There are many who have been shaken by the vision of their own mortality and recovered. Geoff is one of only a few who have transformed the experience into a work through which his life-affirming struggle can be shared with others.

Chris Kourakis

Justice, Supreme Court of South Australia

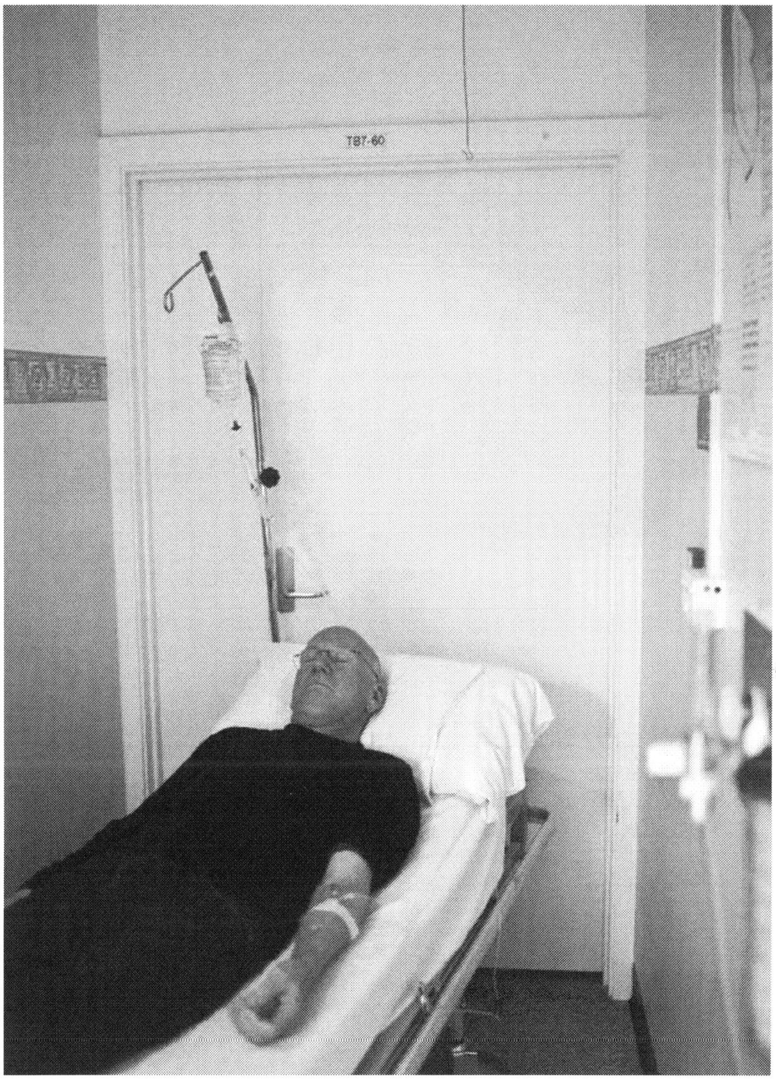

No Small Matter

At the palliative care unit
ten years ago
i watched my father
die of cancer
saw him each day
get smaller
& smaller
& smaller
until he was no bigger
than a leprechaun

i'd joke with him on visits
that we needed to hear his voice
to find him on the sheet
but really—
it was no small matter

i took from him the strength
to challenge myself daily
& since his death
i've swum in the sea twice
a day
& been close enough to
stroke a shark one afternoon
but lucky enough to
have it swim away after we'd
eye-balled each other

i’ve competed too in an 8k run
for cancer awareness
& pink faced & breathless—
been placed third for
my age group

i’ve grunted & groaned
& counted & sweated
through tens of thousands
of sit-ups & push-ups
ached until my stomach
was a washboard

yet still
i got tapped on the
shoulder.

Blue Sky Mornings

I remember being five years old
& walking up & down
the white quartz driveway
of our family home in Copley St
dragging on a Rothmans Plain

i was often up at 5am on those
summer mornings
tip-toeing over the floorboards
& being careful not to let the
screen door slap as i'd creep
out to dad's cream FX Holden
to sneak a smoke out of
the red soft pack he'd left on
the front bench seat

i'd walk the driveway then—
& practise doing the drawback
feeling dizzy at times
but somehow enjoying it
& i might do the
Chinese drawback too—
feeling the smoke drift up my
nostrils
& i remember blowing
smoke rings into perfect blue
sky mornings

looking up at the apricots
at the end of the driveway—
& sometimes hearing them fall
& seeing white cling peaches
still setting on the tree
& the corn already high enough
to hide a boy like me

but i was big enough to work
& even then i knew
i wanted to be a working man

those mornings i'd listen for
the jingle of empty bottles
& the clip-clop of hooves
on our unmade street
knowing that Lennie Sugars
the milky was coming
& i'd butt my smoke into
the red clay soil & bolt out
to meet him

i'd spend the next two hours
placing pints on front verandas—
hearing the clink of empties
from the back of the cart as the
horse worked his way towards
Lennie's low whistle
i remember too—
my forefinger & index finger

greasy from the residue of
so many poorly washed empties
i'd picked up
but over the next fifty years & more—
i'd pick up more than just
greasy bottles

there were sixty to eighty cigarettes
a day for fifteen years
& over twenty half coronas
for another ten
& lots of five paper joints
too

& i'd pick up solvents & sealants
& stains & paints & fluxes
& fluids with peculiar smells
working through twelve hour
days on building sites in blinding sun
with no UV protection

& yet no one can tell me with any
authority
just how i got cancer.

Counting

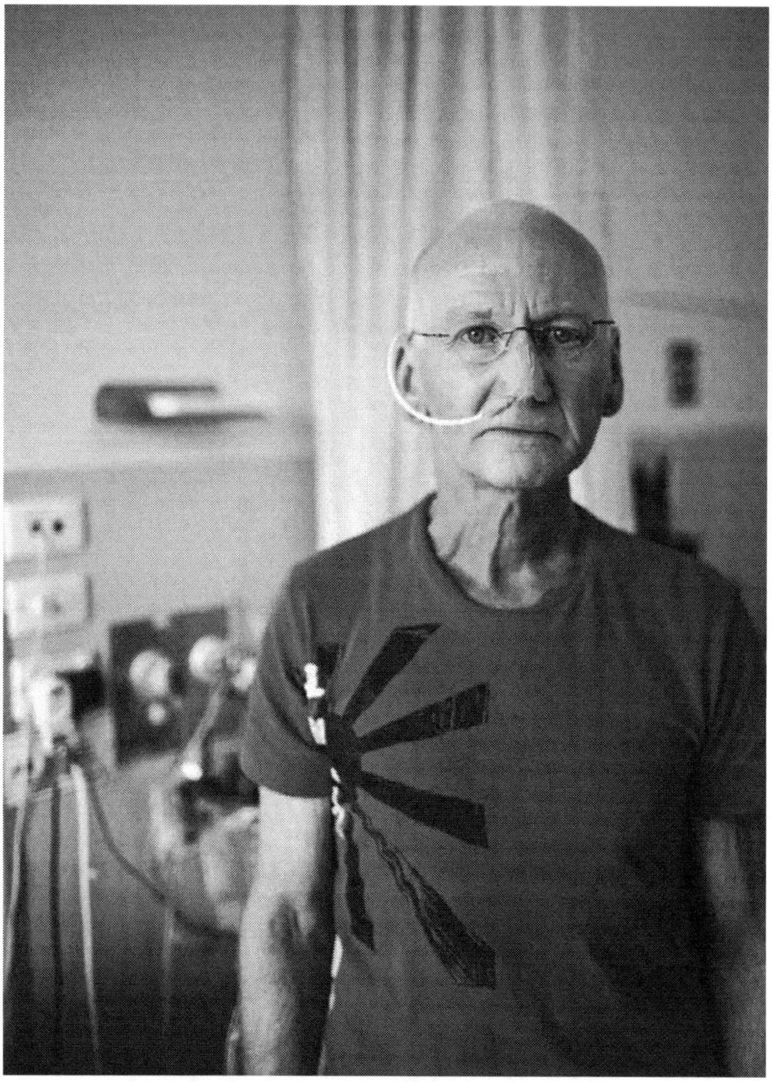

Twenty years ago
when i was feeling
utterly invincible
my first wife's
new partner

Drunken Duncan—
when nearing the bottom
of a cask of white
told me his worst
nightmare was looking
out at his own funeral
& seeing only six
or seven people

i laughed at him
& his blood-shot
blue eyes watered a little

a week after waking one
morning with a lump
in my throat
i was admitted
to a third floor ward

wired up to electronic
gadgets & hooked up to lines
of steroids & painkillers
i found myself
far too wired to sleep

as i looked out before dawn
through double glazed
windows
the distant suburban lights
winked at me

my thoughts then were of
fairyland
& distant people

i started counting.

The Calling

When i was tipped out
of the ward to go home
i hadn't had a chance
to ask doctors if any limits
should apply to my daily life

for over ten years throughout
summers
i'd swum a kilometre
along the shoreline every day
but walking down to the beach
that first morning
i felt scared
not knowing any boundaries

as i trod through the soft sand
i thought about the little
cancer cells eating away at my
decayed throat
& the palm of my hand
felt warm against the bulging
tumour
it was then i wondered if my
raised heart rate would pump
those little critters right through
my body
& scatter cancers everywhere

as i waded into the water i wasn't
looking for sharks
but i felt i was being circled
by something far more sinister
& i decided i couldn't risk it

but still i waded out until the water
felt cool around my throat
& with my mouth barely
above the lapping water
i started to wade the
shoreline

i travelled nearly a kilometre
carefully moving forward—
slow but steady
all the while speaking to the
cancer
i'm here i told it
i'm here to tell you
i'm going to fight you every inch
of the way
you won't beat me
i kept calling
i'm here
i'm here
i'm here.

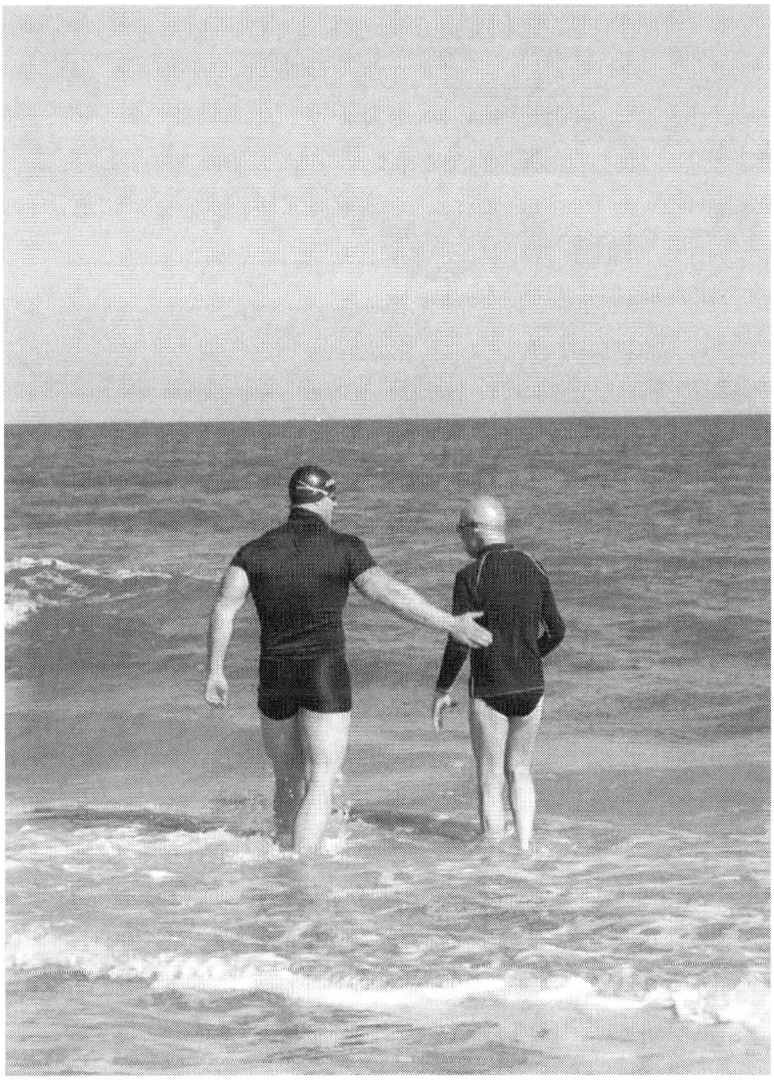

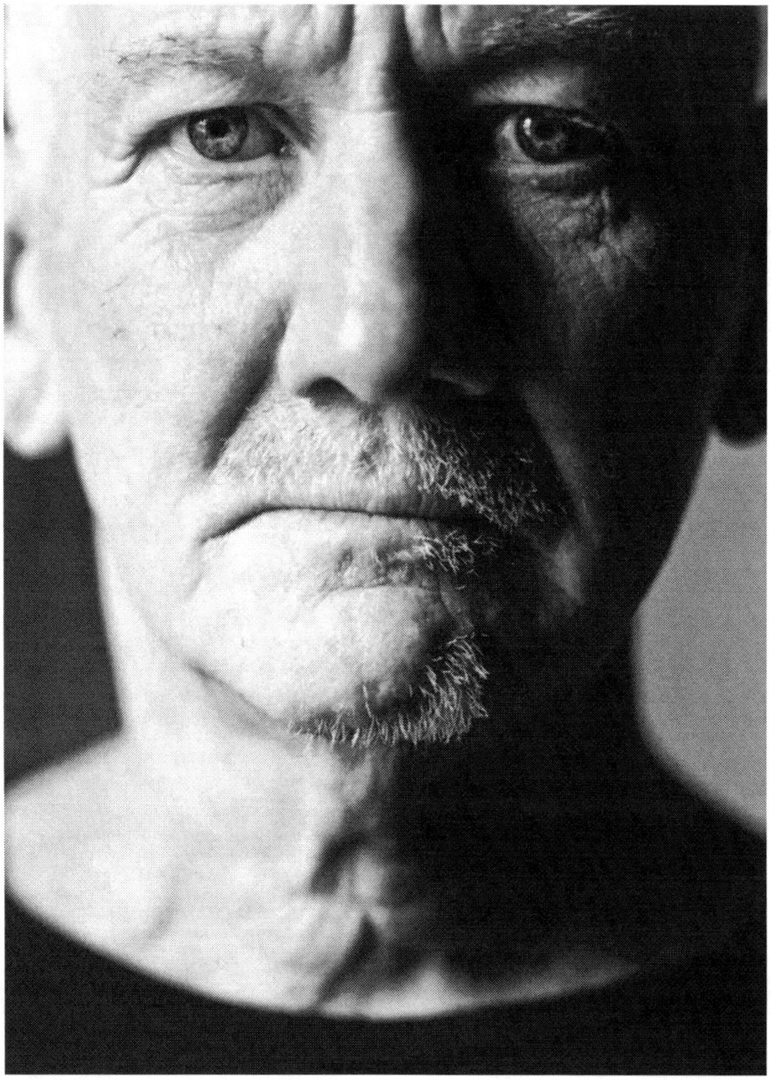

A Long Way from Lourdes

For Sister Judith Redden, AO

As a long lapsed Catholic
i live with my doubt
remembering all too often
when i was under six years of age
being shown no mercy
by the thickness of the leather strap
driving home a nun's message

now that i'm facing procedures for
cancer at nearly sixty
a principal nun (a principled nun)
has sent home a 40ml bottle
of holy water from Lourdes
with my sixteen year old daughter

i am scheduled for two operations
a week apart

i sip half the contents before each
procedure

my agnostic editor thinks i'm mad.

The Seventh Doctor

The first doctor i saw was my
local GP
he said i had the flu
& the lump in my neck
was bunched up muscle
he told me to go home—
drink plenty of water
& eat Panadeine Forte & Valium

i saw him again five days later
& told him i'd hardly slept
he sent me home once more
& told me to add sleeping tablets
to the mix

two days later when i was
dangerously dizzy
like dad when he was drunk
& disorderly
i drove myself to the public
hospital

some people said to me later
i was silly & should have
called an ambulance
but i'm not in the ambulance
fund

& i didn’t have money for a
taxi
& i’m an independent
bastard too

after a near side-swipe to
a neighbour’s car just
a hundred metres from home
i sat up pretty quick—
thinking of the thickness of a coat
of paint
& i rolled the windows down
& caught the breeze
it was a slow five k drive

after a few minutes in the emergency
waiting room i thought i was going
to fall off the chair
so i asked to lie on a
stretcher
a man with a grey flecked beard
came across & spoke
he told me they were reserved for
sick people & i should stay in my chair
i told him he’d be sick if he didn’t
wheel the stretcher over for me NOW

after i’d lain down he leaned over me
& said
you’ll have to get off if anyone

comes in who really needs it
i suggested he'd better be able to
fight if he thought i'd be getting off

it only took another five hours & i was
moved in to see the second doctor
when he saw how awkward i was—
& noticed how long it took me to sit
upright
& saw i hadn't shaved for a week—
& heard my slurred speech
he folded his arms & told me to go
home have a sleep & go back & see
that first doctor

i told him to get fucked
met his eyes—
& said that if he didn't look at me
properly
i'd spread him over the floor

after a look & a feel he sent me
for a cat scan

when i returned he said
i've called in a specialist—
you might have to wait for an hour
or so because he's coming from
another hospital

when i saw the third doctor he said
you are very sick—
you have an infected abscess
& it’s very close to the voice box
you’ll need to go into a bed
upstairs
you may need an operation
in the morning

when they got me installed upstairs
i saw the fourth doctor
he said—
you’d better prepare yourself
this could be the big c

i thought i’d already met the big c
when i saw that second doctor

in the morning i met the fifth doctor
a woman—
who one day later told me i did have
cancer
but the way she told me
made me think she was the big c
the lady doctor told me to go
home she said they’d ring me
with a time to go to another hospital
to see another doctor

after a week when no one had rung

i rang the hospital

i spoke to a sixth doctor who told me
they never said they would ring me
he said i was confused—
& that i should wait for a phone call
or a letter

i told the sixth doctor that maybe
he was confused
i said i remembered what
i'd been told

he said
no you are confused
we will tell you when we want to see
you
& we'll do that by letter or phone—
whatever suits us best
if you don't like it—
you know what to do
you can go private & call the tune
& have doctors suit your timetable

i reminded the sixth doctor
i was a public patient & had no
private cover
but i told him too i was
an old fashioned bloke

i said
i'll keep an eye on the letterbox
& an ear out for the phone
but i'll go outside every hour
& check the roof for homing pigeons
so feel free to send your instructions
by carrier pigeon
i've got a long ladder & a seventeen
foot high wall & i feel quite confident
i can climb the ladder & open up the
metal band & retrieve any messages
you might like to send
i'm happy to use the old technology—
or the new i'll leave it up to you

the sixth doctor suggested we end the call

with respect i said
maybe i am confused & i don't really
have cancer
can you confirm that i actually do
have cancer

yes he replied you do

& can you confirm that i did have an
ultra sound examination

yes he replied you did
& while i freely admit i don't have much

medical knowledge
i do have a good understanding
of the nuances of language & speech
& i do believe when the ultra sound
examination was carried out
there was a good deal of surprise in
the voices of the five or six people
behind me in that darkened room
would you agree on that point

yes he replied i agree

& while i don't want to appear pedantic
would you agree that four or perhaps
even five biopsy samples were removed
during that examination
i'm sure i do remember the pull on the
flesh
& i'm sure i heard instructions
on how deep to go one point five
centimetetres two centimetres
etcetera etcetera
i mean i won't argue on the number
of biopsies or the depth of the needles
it's the procedure i'm referring to—
would you agree that i did in fact have several
biopsy samples taken

yes he replied i agree
well thank you i said

i'll keep an eye on the letterbox
an ear out for the phone
& i'll check the roof hourly
thank you doctor for your decency
your humanity
& your kindness

& we both hung up

after a few more weeks i got to meet
the seventh doctor a surgeon
a decent bloke who showed me
decency & got it in return
he explained my condition
in a language i could understand
his handshake was as solid as
his eye contact & i liked his style

the seventh doctor had me lie on the
operating table for a biopsy
on my tongue because they couldn't
locate my primary
the cancer in my neck was a secondary

on the day of the op he & his team all wore
blue overalls white gumboots
caps & masks
they looked like concrete finishers
on a building site
but their hands were soft & their vowels

were rounded

before i was sent off to sleep
the seventh doctor talked to me
about painting
& Robert Hannaford—
& poetry & art as therapy
he sure didn't sound like
a concrete finisher

when i awoke i was put into a ward of
other old men who coughed all night
& kept one another awake
& when the screen curtains were
drawn in the morning
i asked the man alongside me
if he'd like a Rothmans Plain

in his morning haze he couldn't fathom
my joke

later that morning i met a tribe of surgical
doctors who told me to go home
my results would take five days
to process

but at six o'clock that night i had
to go back
the abscess had started to swell
again

& i met doctor eight

he arranged my re-admission & i was
given a different bed in the same ward
& dripped with antibiotics
when i awoke in the morning my chin
was a mass of sores
& my bottom lip looked as though
it had been pumped with botox

doctors nine & ten came to see me after
i asked the nurse to get me a doctor
but they were completely baffled

they didn't seem to be much older than
my teenage daughter
& when they started mentioning the
possibility of a staf infection
the nurse looked really alarmed

doctor nine suggested to doctor ten
they should go & look in their books to
see if they could identify the problem

when they left i told the nurse i'd like
to see a grown-up doctor
i was scared & so was she

when she came back with doctor eleven
she told him she'd like to move me from

the ward to a private room

doctor eleven said he didn't deem that
necessary
he suggested it was maybe school sores
i suggested it might be cold sores
but doctor eleven couldn't agree

i said i wanted to see a specialist
it was a teaching hospital
& they must have someone capable of
an accurate diagnosis

by the time doctor twelve arrived the
nurse had panicked & moved me to
a private room
i repeated to doctor twelve
i thought it might be cold sores due to
stress
but he couldn't agree either

the following morning a tribe of surgical
doctors looked at me
& no one seemed too sure

it was then that doctor thirteen came
to my bedside & cut the heads off
some of the pustules & swabbed me

days later when the results finally arrived

the spread had really increased
& the lip grown larger
& i did in fact have cold sores—
but they called it herpes simplex virus

two days later they sent me home
with a bottle of condy's crystals
& packets of anti viral tabs

about two weeks further down the track
i met doctor fourteen a dental doctor
the split corners of my mouth were
still healing but she needed to inspect my
gums & teeth before my neck dissection
the next day
i asked her to be careful said i
didn't have a big mouth
(although i'm sure some doctors
[& others] would dispute that)
but she treated me with care—
stating that i did have a small opening
(& though i enjoy puns i said nothing)
her advice was to get a tube of
Daktarin cream & use it overnight
but more importantly—
to smear it over the corners of my mouth
just prior to the operation
she said it would be likely to stop
any cold sores from coming back
& she was right

that next morning i saw doctor seven
again in the same operating theatre
he had his tribe of surgical doctors to
back him up along with two anaesthetists
& a few nurses
as i was wheeled in
my eyes scanned for familiar faces
doctor eight was smiling broadly
so i winked at him
he understood my style & his smile
broadened

a couple of days later doctor eight
told me the surgical team had read
some of my poetry aloud as i was going
off
that was doctor seven's idea

doctor eight said they'd stopped because
some of it seemed a little 'R' rated
he said that after some of my lines
were read he remembered hearing me read
when he was a teenager at St Peter's College
i remarked that it must have been
during Ray Stanley's reign
when the school was a bit more liberal—
& more than just one voice was heard

he laughed at that
& i laughed too

i wasn't laughing when i woke up from
the neck dissection though
it was 5:20pm when i sighted the clock
in the intensive care unit & i was feeling
cranky
squinting wondering where my glasses
were & trying to calculate how long i'd been
lying there & did they know i was awake
at 7:30pm they wheeled me back to the ward
the same one i'd been in before but again—
a different berth

& there to greet me was my girlfriend
& my youngest son Paul
we counted backwards & calculated
it must have been a long operation
they said the wound looked like i'd
been carved up with a broken flagon
they said a bottle would have been
far too small they said it looked scary—
& because i couldn't see
what my visitors saw
i asked a nurse for a mirror

it scared me too

by 9pm though i was asking for food
as much to my own surprise as that of
my visitors
but the swallowing wasn't fun

doctor seven had cut me from the bottom
of my left earlobe
to the top of my collarbone
then curled around & up to my adam's apple
it was a cut as big as a baling hook
& with its thirty metal staples
it looked almost as shiny & nearly as
dangerous

he'd performed his surgery on Holy Thursday
20th March 2008
& with the neck muscle removed he'd
left a hole but he'd taken the tumour too
(intact we hope) & with two previous
infections it had been quite a messy job
he was back at my bedside on Good Friday
morning away from his own four kids
explaining that i'd gone through the
easy part of the treatment
that the chemo & the radiation were
to come in about six weeks
after the wound had healed

he told me to go home & get into
the full cream milk the banana smoothies
all the chocolate i could eat & anything else
that took my fancy & was fattening
to get some weight on because i'd sure
as hell get it stripped off in six weeks time
he told me too that my voice box had been

welded to the tumour
that he’d had to cut it free & there’d
been some nerve damage & my voice mightn’t
improve a lot on what i had at that point
but i was still talking
& i was still listening
grateful to have doctor seven on my side

it was a good Friday to get that news
i lay in bed eating Easter eggs—
silver paper & cellophane
surrounding me
chocolate sliding down my throat.

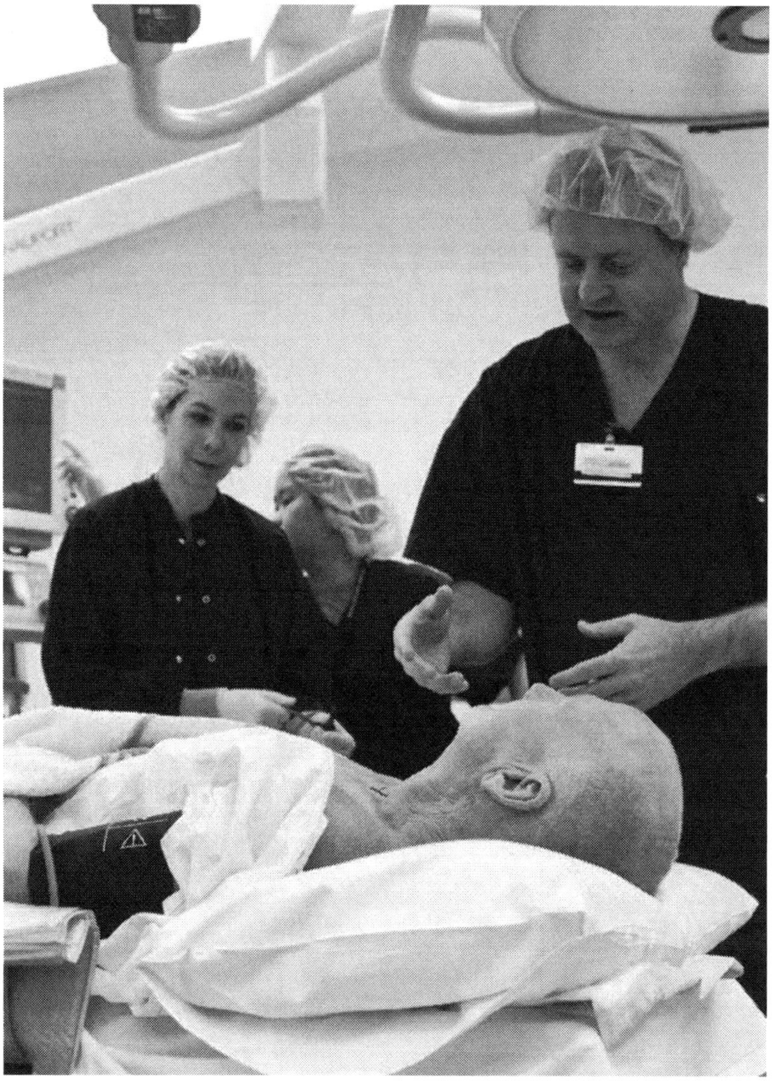

Maybe

In the Head & Neck ward
most of us blokes are fifty plus
old Marlboro men
on Alpine white beds
now that's Kool

& i'll give you the Drum
it could well be Winfield
Reds on the right
& Blues on the left
(geez that looks like Blue
in bed seven
hasn't he lost some weight)
& where is Paul Hogan
when we really need a laugh

post op now with stapled
throats after our neck dissections

maybe it'll hurt too much

maybe there's nothing much
to laugh at anymore

maybe now the laugh's
on us.

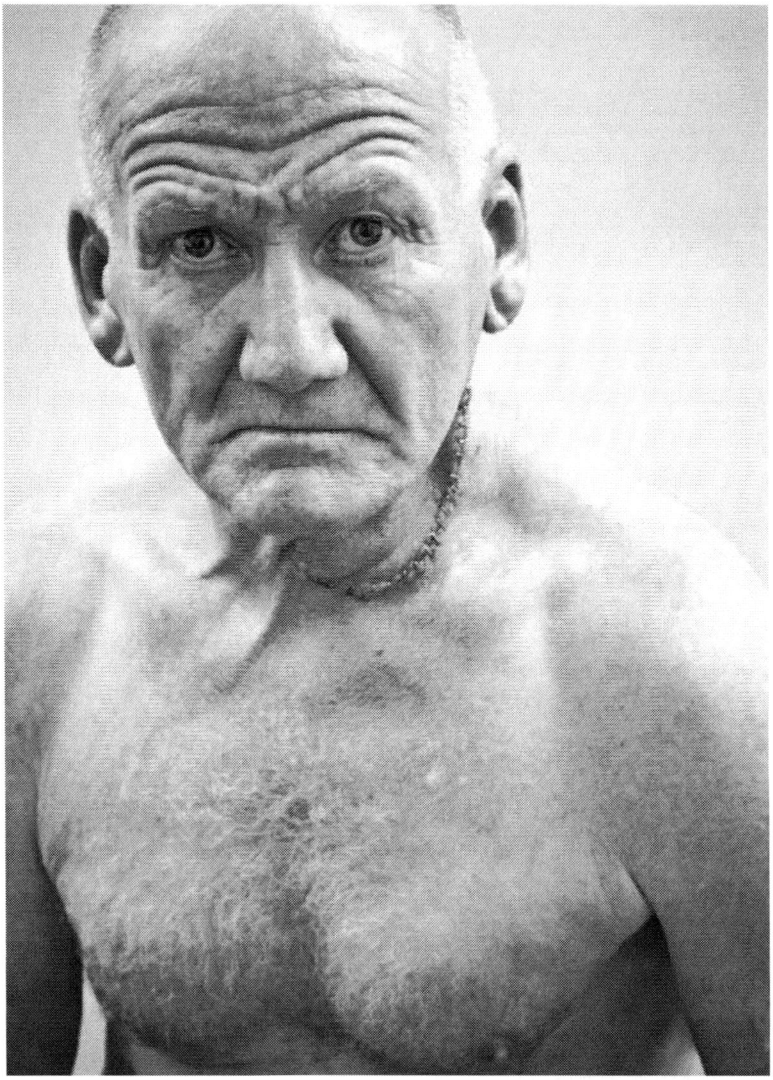

Finding Myself

At fifty plus the morning shave
was invariably something
i did from a distance

standing in the shower alcove
three metres across the bathroom
from the mirror
to squint at a rough
reflection of my father

confident that i knew the contours
of my face & neck
always careful to avoid
the sebaceous cyst below
my right earlobe
the one that always proved
a mountain could be made
out of a molehill if i passed
over it with the triple blade
a touch too heavy

always having to make sure
the tiny bump of a scar
below my lip didn't get too
close & turn the shaving cream
red
& cause me to snarl & swear

but now at fifty-eight with a
major neck dissection
done two weeks ago
the left side of my neck
muscle removed
the thirty metal staples gone—
the scar starting to heal
i find myself frosting the
mirror with my own breath
my cheeks now sallow & slack
after surgery
still too tentative
(even with my glasses on)
to sweep away the morning
stubble

& once again i'm a young boy
my strokes deliberate & planned

while in the mirror
my father's blue eyes squint—
& watch every move.

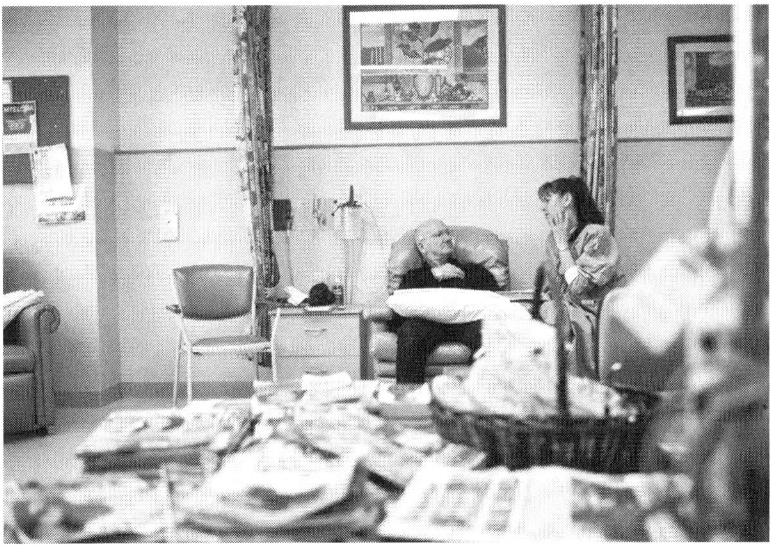

Time Bomb

On my first day of chemo
i didn't know what to expect

Lisa my appointed nurse
put a drip into my right hand
& told me there was about
four & a half litres to go in

the machine pumped in
a saline solution hanging in a clear
plastic bag on a chrome stand

the Baxter pump ticked
with monotonous regularity

when Lisa hung the black bag
marked
Caution: Cytotoxic
Handle with gloves
i knew i had the real deal

six patients all sat patiently
taking in their chemo

apart from the ticking—
the room was filled with
our combined silences

after some minutes a woman spoke—
it sounds like a time bomb
going off

it is i whispered *it is.*

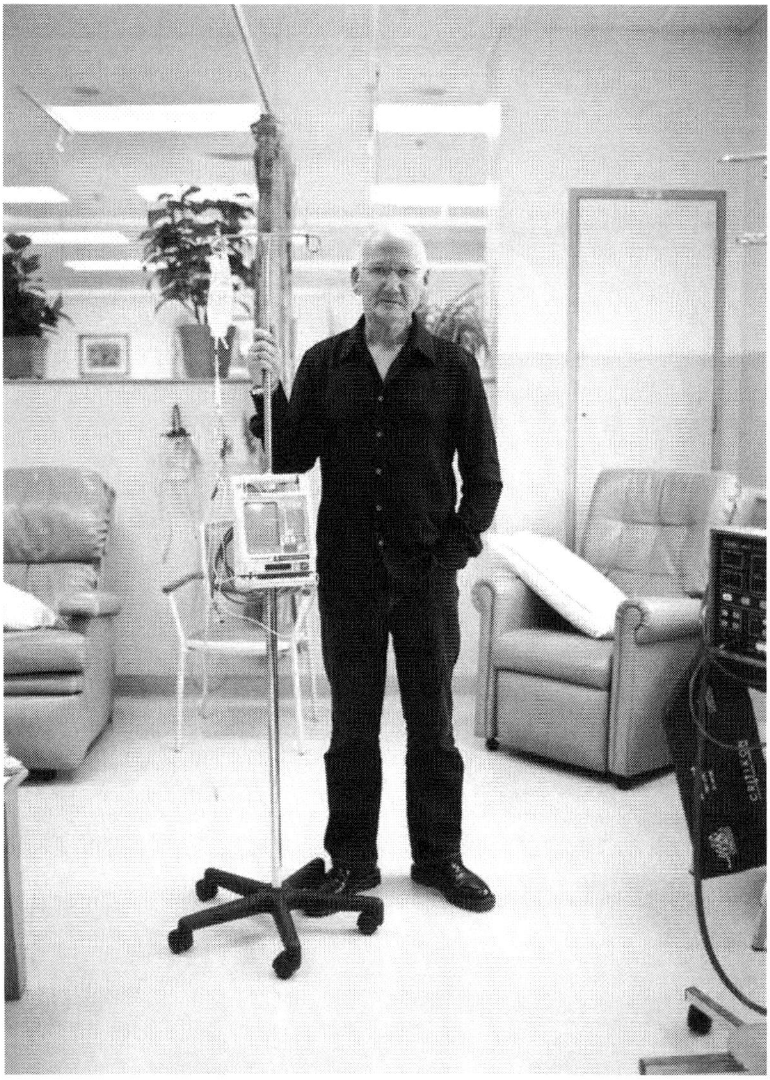

Round One

About five hours into taking
my first dose of chemo
i called the nurse over
& said *excuse me Lisa*
but my Jelco is stinging

she looked down at the back
of my hand & said
look—
you've bent the stem

i'd had about four litres
of saline & chemicals
pumped into me throughout
the day
& i'd been backwards
& forwards to the toilet
many times

she straightened the stem
& strapped me with a
clear plastic dressing

then she said with a hint
of menace
don't move so much

i replied drily
they never said that to
Muhammad Ali

how do you know? she replied

i'm an old fighter i told her

she shook her head & rolled her eyes.

Hospital Ship

In the morning—
after the blinds were drawn
the man opposite
commented on what
a stormy night it'd been

as i gazed out of the windows
i told him the waves had been
crashing over the wheelhouse
overnight
i said it was good that
the ship was stable & had
withstood the storm
i suggested it certainly
must have a deep keel

he nodded agreement
then asked if i'd been on
this ship before

i told him i usually sailed Sitmar
but that i'd been with this mob
on a few voyages

after breakfast
as i was packing my case—
i told him i was leaving the ship

where are you going? he asked

Buenos Aries i replied
i'm joining another cruise

have you got your passport? he asked

yes i've got my passport
& my visa too
all is under control—
i'll be fine

when the nurse signalled that
i was being moved to another
room
i nodded to him & said
bon voyage Claude
enjoy your trip

i can still see him waving.

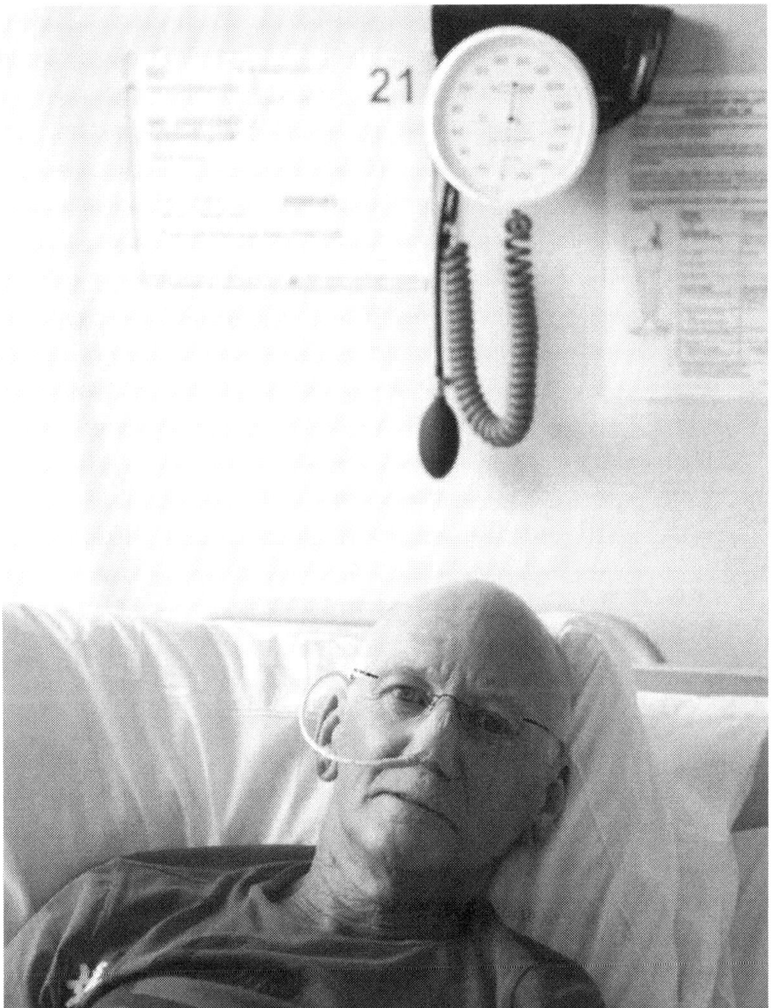
21

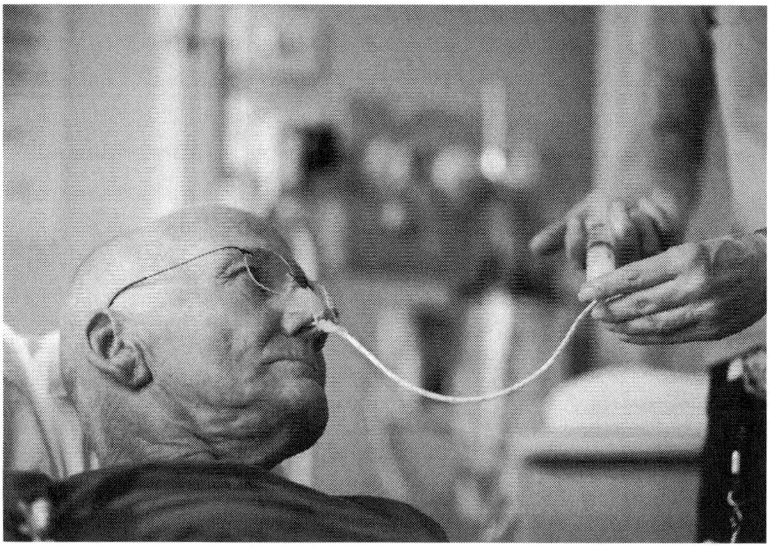

Night Moves

Halfway through the chemo
& the radio
when i was unable to eat
& had the naso gastric tube
poked up my nostril & into my
stomach
when my temp was
hovering around 40C
i found myself
back in hospital
for a further three weeks

most nights my own nausea
kept me awake
along with the snores
of other old men around me
some nights it was the man
opposite me who kept calling
Josephine
Josephine
Josephine
until the nurses came with their
torches & quietened him
assuring him he was in hospital
& not at home

it was on the tenth night of that

sleep deprived period when i
finally snapped
it was the anniversary of my
brother's sudden death just
three years earlier

i was keen to sleep & dream
of Brian
but they'd parked me
alongside an old man with
dementia

sometime after midnight he
shut up long enough for me to
fall asleep

at 2:30am though he rose
from his cot—
trying to climb up
& over the side rails
when he woke me
he didn't speak a word
of English & was yelling
at the nurses in Croatian
& he went on
& on
& on

at 3:30am i rang my bell & asked
for a couple of sleeping tablets

& some pain relief

the old man was still going
when the nurses returned with
the controlled drug for me
as they injected me
i said to them softly
if he keeps this up
i'll suffocate him with a pillow

after breakfast
they moved me to a private room.

Day & Night/Night & Day

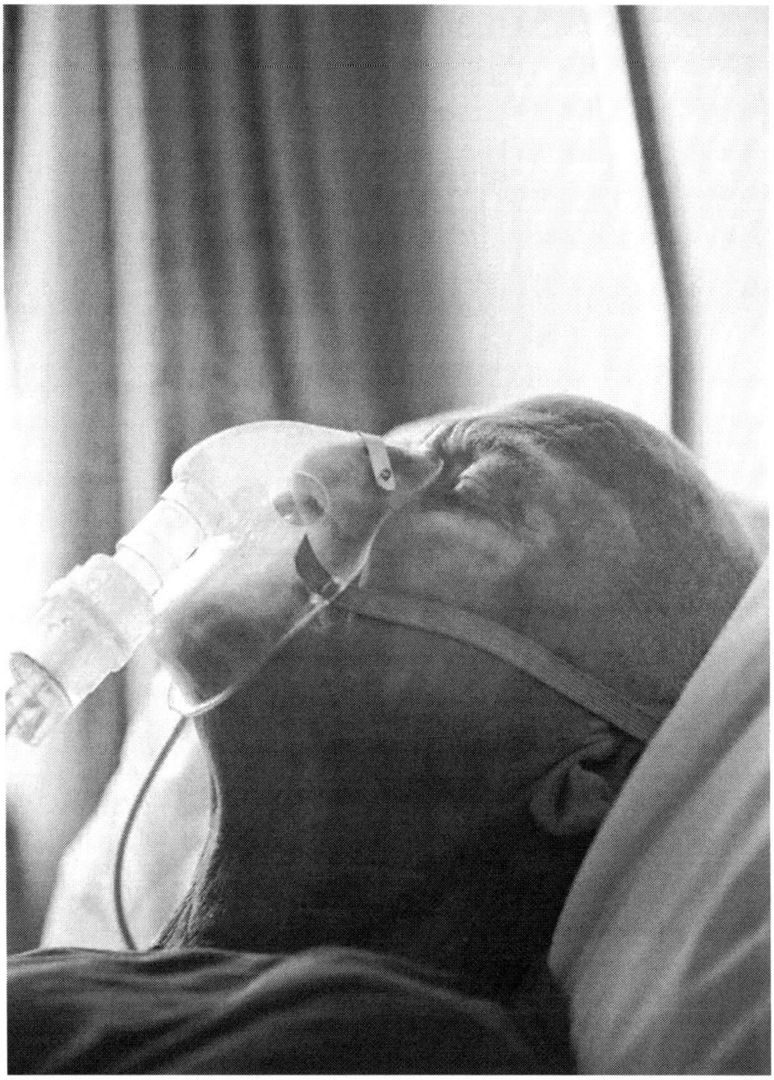

My recovery from chemo & radio
seemed worse than the cancer
at the time
wave after wave of nausea
would have me crawling around

the bed on my hands & knees
trying to vomit—
but i was never quite able
to get there
then explosive action in
the toilet
& back to bed again for
more gut wrenching pain
my tongue burning from
the radiation
ulcers raging through my
mouth
& the creamy phlegm
flowing freely as yet another
box of tissues hit the bin

day & night it went on
night & day

sometimes a snatched hour
of sleep if i was lucky

more than likely out of bed
at 2am for my four hourly ritual
gargle soda water
& follow up with Difflam
& follow up with Curacept
& follow up with Amethocaine
& back to bed—
& still no sleep to follow

lying in the half light
of the ward
my bottles of mouthwash
silhouetted
lined up like soldiers
on the bedside table
while i'd swipe another
tissue to wrap another
mouthful of phlegm

all the while watching the
clock through the early hours
waiting on a 6am nebuliser

i needed to breathe.

Ticket to Ride

The radiation ritual
ran for six weeks
daily i'd lie
on my back on the x-ray
bench
a personal moulded
mask of plastic mesh
encasing my head & shoulders
allowing me to be
rigidly clipped down to the
bench

in that dimly lit room
i'd listen to the assistants
either side of me as they'd
line up their laser beams
to match the grid of my mask
& i'd shuffle up—
or down or left or right
as directed

then with my eyes closed tight
& my mouth muffled
i'd begin to feel
claustrophobic

& the voice of an

assistant would soothe me
telling me to wave my arm
if it got too much
& they'd retreat
to monitor me on a closed
circuit TV

it was then i'd begin to imagine
i was a jet pilot on a trip
i'd allow myself to believe
the whirring of the x-ray was
a jet engine
& the grinding & the clanking
were the wheels retracting
after take off & on landing

each trip was similar
but different too—
some of my voyages were
disturbed mid flight by
the return of the assistants
to make adjustments
& i'd locate these in my
mind as refuelling points

& as much as i hated this
daily ritual
i believed every flight
i took
could be my ticket home.

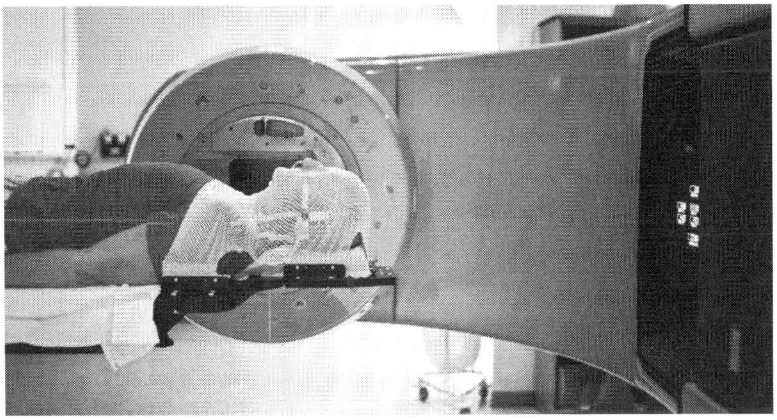

Onto the Spin Cycle

I've started waltzing with
jack dancer
gliding—
in a slow spin cycle
while trying
to maintain my balance

i've had to walk away from
twelve months paid work
cancel my ninth consecutive
tour of Tasmania
knock-back a trip to New York
& Toronto
learn to survive on a
disability support pension
& use tricks like drip feeding
the fuel tank for doctor's visits

at the same time i've had to cop
a fifty dollar rate hike from my
landlord
buy a two hundred dollar
electric razor because blades
are banned on radiotherapy
patients

find another four hundred

& fifty for spectacles with
titanium frames
my *D & G* plastic frames
squeezed my scalp too tight
too hard too painfully—
after head & neck surgery

& just when i thought i could see
where i was heading again
i had my hand in my pocket
to find another two hundred
for a microwave oven
the same oven i'd avoided
owning for twenty odd years
because of the threat
of radiation leakage
but now—
weakened from my intake of chemo
& my daily radiation therapy
i'm unable to stand around
& peel & chop & slice & cook
i need to quickly heat the
frozen meals that are stacked
in my freezer

& though my cancer arrived
in a heat wave
it's winter now as i face six
weeks of chemo

& the oil heater spins the disc
on my electricity meter
& spins
& spins

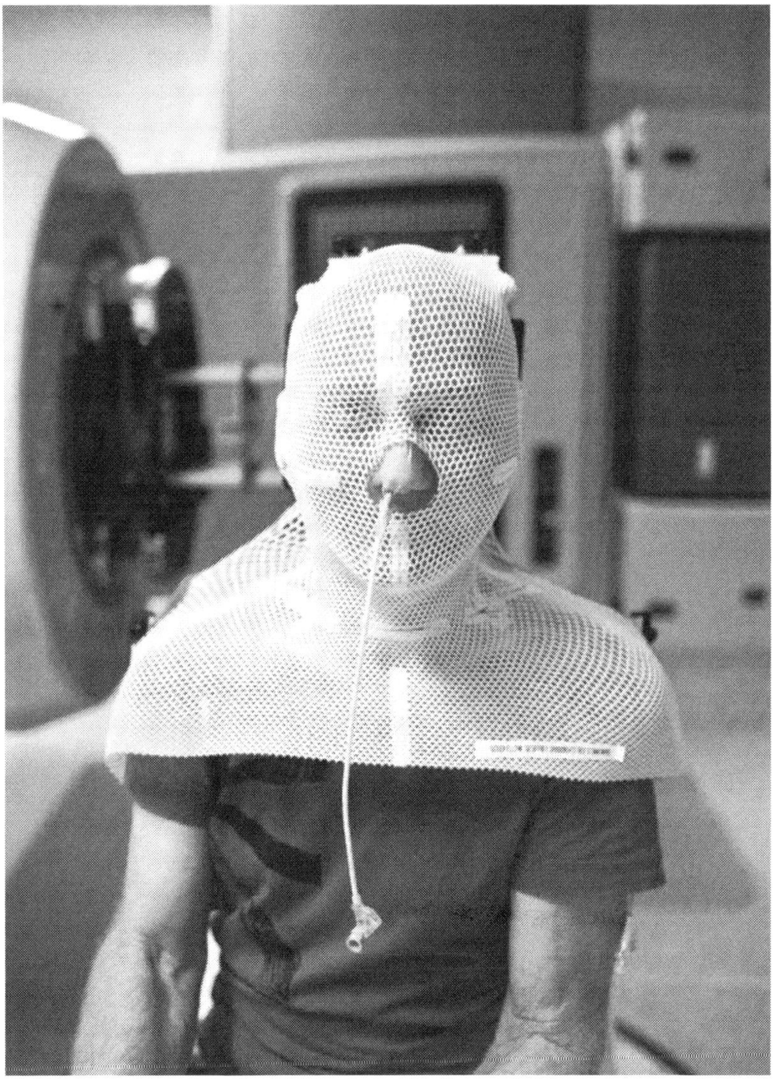

Begging Bowl

Hi she said *i'm the dietician*
& she gave me a sly smile
& skidded a low armchair
across the hospital vinyl
to a screeching halt alongside
my bed

we need to get some weight
on you while you're here
now i see you're
drinking soda water
we can start with that—
there's no calories in soda water
so you'd be best to change
to lemonade a couple of
bottles a day will soon start
to make a difference

listen i said *i've had radiotherapy*
i can't have any of my
lower teeth removed ever again—
& i'd really like to be able to keep
my top teeth too
i don't want to have sticky
sugary teeth so i'll stay with the
soda water which works well as
a mouthwash as i'm still dealing

with a bit of mucositis

it's the volume of food i'm
being fed here that's half my problem
at home i'd have three to four
times as much porridge as i got
in my bowl this morning
i'd be happy if you gave me
two bowls tomorrow
that would make a big difference
for me

well she said
how about we give you a
slice of bread or perhaps even toast
instead?

that's no good i replied
i don't have salivary glands
so i can't eat bread or toast or pastries
but an extra bowl of porridge
would be great

well she said
how about we give you
an egg or even a couple of eggs?

that's no good either i told her
eggs are too sticky & get caught
in my throat

but an extra bowl of porridge
would just slide down my throat

well she said
we can't actually give you an
extra bowl of porridge
we really need to supplement you
with something else

i looked at her in amazement
you're terminated i said—
& i turned away & picked up
the newspaper & read a headline

she sat there unmoved

i took a deep breath
shot another look at her
& repeated myself

she still sat there unmoved

i took yet another deep breath
threw the newspaper back
on the bed & barked
you're terminated
you've got the sack
go away fuck off
do you understand me now
go away & annoy someone else

but don't annoy me anymore

she skittered across the room

in the morning i had two bowls.

After Effects

Pre cancer
i usually ate light rye bread
throughout the working week

winter weekends
it would likely be sourdough—
or a crusty wood bake oven
or sometimes a ciabatta
if my daughter had her way

throughout summer it was always
Turkish bread
light & fluffy like the clouds—
& a Danish pastry as a treat
to follow a full breakfast at Lucias
Saturday mornings

now six months after surgery—
with my radiation complete
my salivary glands are all
burnt out
my mouth is as dry as
a cardboard box
my tongue feels like it's been
scraped with a vegetable peeler

& my mouth ulcers still

make sure i wake several times
throughout the night

like now it's 3:42am
& i'm wondering what my weight
will be at 7:00 when i usually rise
yesterday it was 67.6kg—
400 grams up on my minimum
struck earlier this week
a far call from the 82kg
i weighed this time last year

there'll be no bread with my
breakfast this morning
or pastries or cake—
& not tomorrow either
or on any other day

each mouthful now
turns into a walnut shape
of stodge within minutes

the after effects of radiation
are very hard to swallow.

Another Fight

On Friday 29 August 1968
i fought Lou Cecere in a prelim
Welterweight bout over 4 threes
at the Thebarton Town Hall

Lou was coming off a string of
early knockouts
& the bloke could hit—
i'd seen his last fight in Mildura
just weeks earlier

at eighteen though
nothing phased me—
i felt cocky & invincible
thought i could dead-set
knock him out
but without any training
i knew i'd have to be quick

when the bell rang we touched
gloves & i rushed him
spearing him with double
straight lefts & a right cross
working those lefts & trying
to position his head

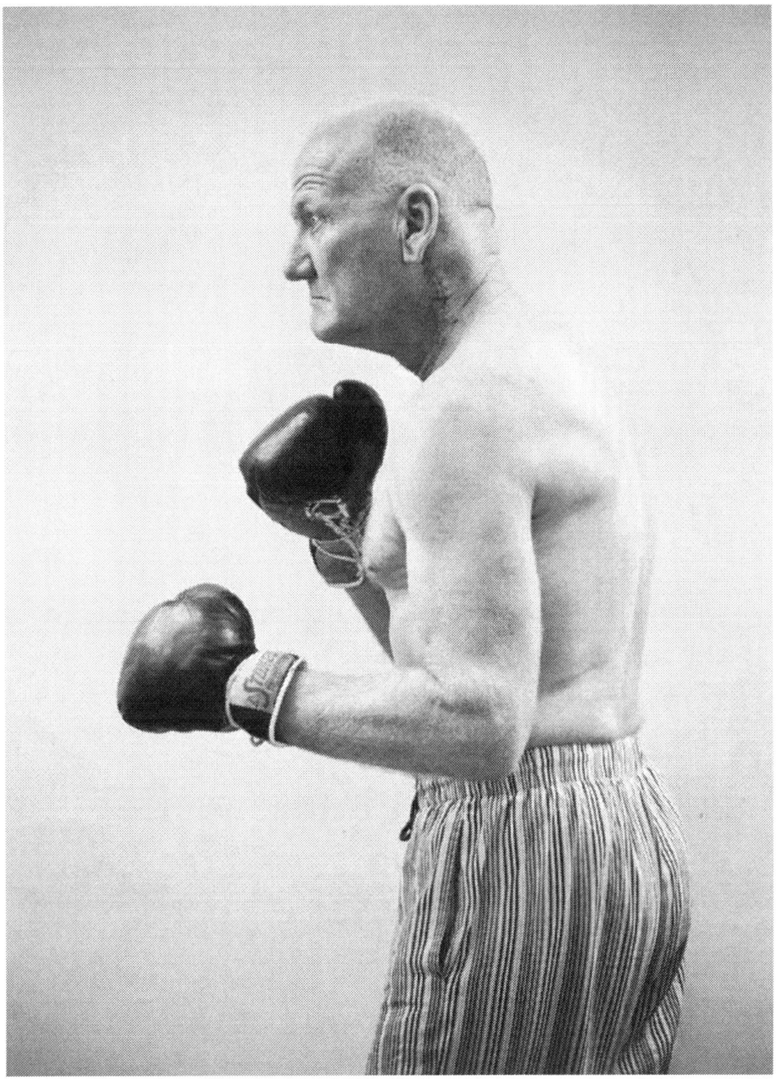

towards the end of that first round
i could see his knees start to
buckle
i've got him
i've got him
i've got him
is what i remember thinking
but my gloves were getting

heavier
& my arms weaker

just before the bell Lou came back
with a flurry of blows & put
me down for an eight count

i've been saved by the bell
i was thinking as i climbed
to one knee
looking for my cornerman

Colin Fox the referee thought the bell
couldn't save me
but he could—
& he waved the fight to an end

in some ways i was disappointed
but i was relieved too—
boxing is a hard earn

Lou & i have stayed close friends
for over forty years now
& when he heard i had
Jack Dancer
he came knocking on my door

climbing my stairs he called out
Geoff Goodfellow's got cancer
well i've got news for cancer

Geoff Goodfellow doesn't run from
anyone
he was silly enough not to run
from me
LOOK OUT CANCER

i think Lou's picked it right too
after six months sparring—
the doctors have me well ahead
on points
but i'm still going for a knockout.

Sip & Squirt

It's been the same routine
for six months now
brush with a no-foam
toothpaste
rinse with an anti-plaque—
& into bed at seven

i'm always too tired to sit up
but i'm far too awake—
to fall asleep

& i lie there sipping
sodawater
or squirting dry mouth gel
onto my tongue & swirling it
around the cheeks of my mouth
trying to relieve the
dryness

my mouth feels like i've been
chewing sticks of chalk
& my tongue looks like
a whiteboard

there's maybe a snatched hour
of sleep
but i'm awake by ten

& up for a pee
then back to bed to
sip & squirt

& i'm up again for a squirt
at two

then back to bed to sip
& squirt
the back of my throat now
dry as a cardboard box
& with some luck i'll
sleep till five

& once again i find myself
lying in the half-light
the back of my throat
feeling like it's been rubbed
with sandpaper
& i lie sipping—
& sipping
& sipping
till i have to get up to pee

i go downstairs for
porridge then
enough for three—
& it's full cream milk
with splashes of cream
& spoons of honey

till it slides down my throat

but within the hour
the chalk
& the whiteboard return

& i continue to sip & squirt.

Triple Digits

For ten years now
i've exercised heavily
at 8am & 5pm each day

to keep myself honest
& to monitor my progress
i've charted my efforts
& religiously recorded
my weights

i've swum from 1200
to 1600 each session
then run hard on
soft beach sand in return

then home to my bedroom
to generally record
200 sit-ups
50 push-ups
& six sets of 20 reps with
7kg dumb-bells

pre-cancer my 2007 records
show a mean average
rising weight of 79.2kg

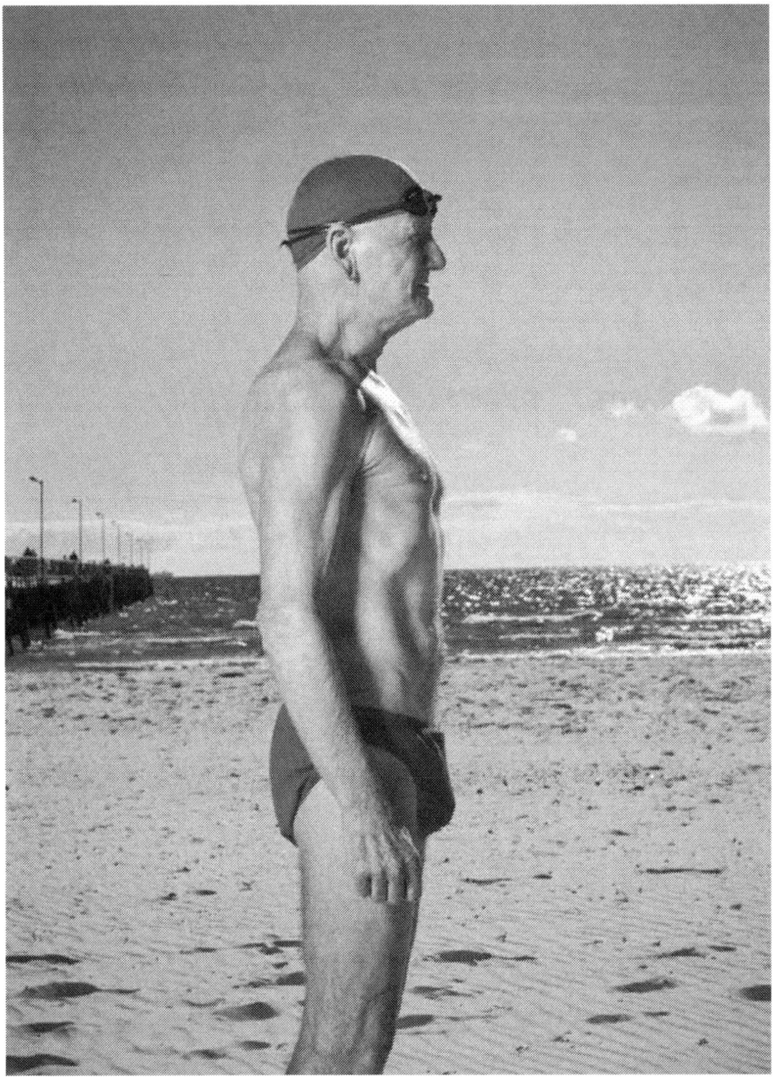

post-op now with my radiation
& chemo complete
the hard earned muscle mass
has been all eaten away
i haven't got
the energy or mental strength
to swim or run or exercise

but habit still causes me to step
onto the scales when i rise

i hit a low point two weeks ago
of 66.2kg
but over the past month
with custards icecreams
& banana smoothies—
i've raised the bar to give me
a mean average of 66.6kg

it's been a devil of a weight
for me to bear.

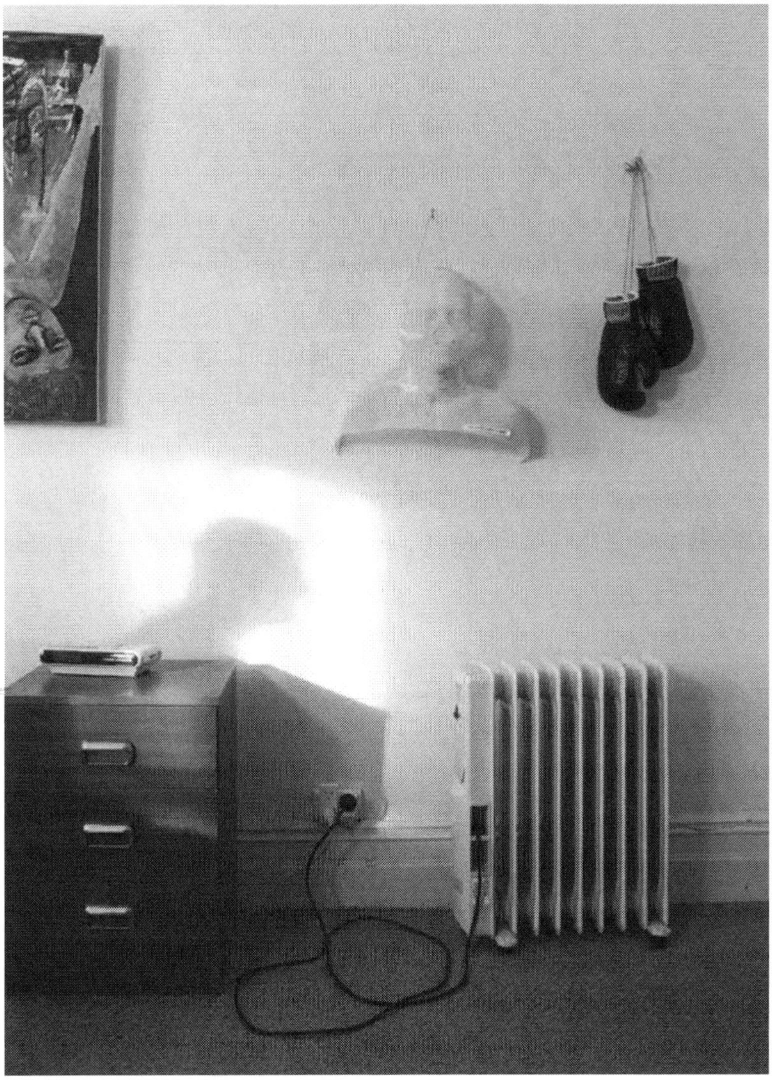

Family History

Like my father
i was born in the first
half of the last century

like his father
(who was born in the last
half of the previous century)
we all smoked over sixty
cigarettes a day

my grandfather died of
throat cancer
two years into the last half
of the last century
(a younger man than me)

my father died of
lung cancer & emphysema
three years short
of this century
(a far older man than me)

i butted out of the cigarette
debate
a decade before the start
of this century

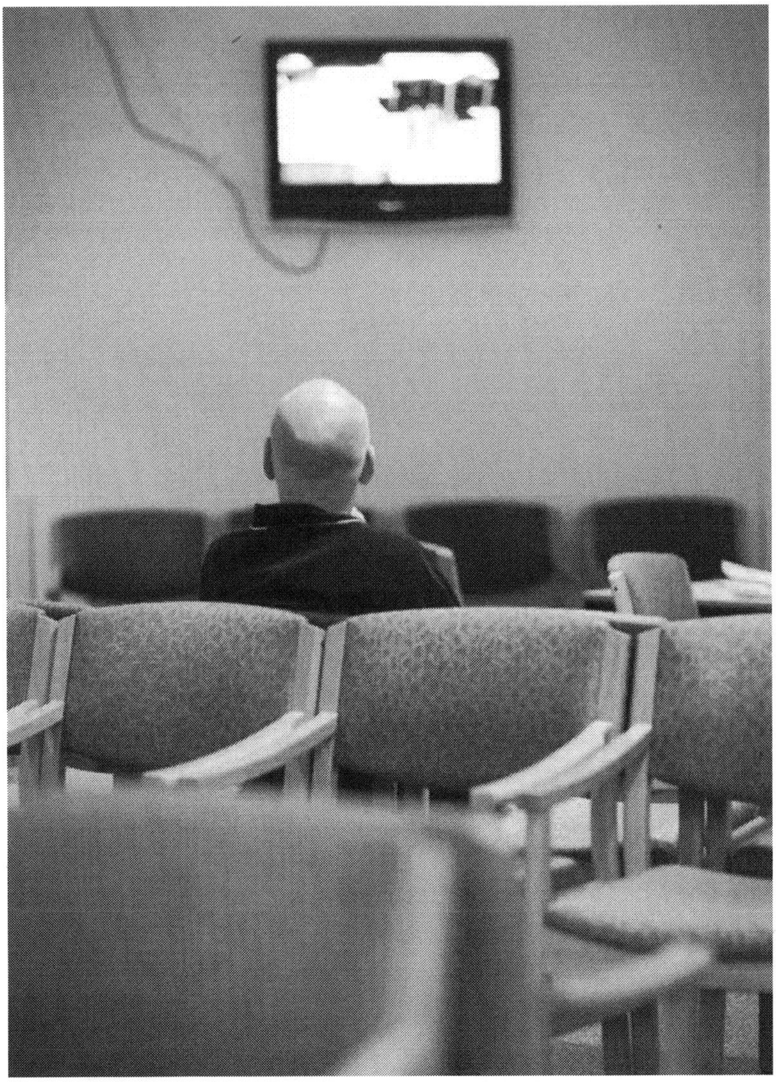

but eight years into
this century
a surgeon had to open
me up & remove a 250g tumour
& the left side of my voice box

i’m hoping now i’ll be able
to see out most of the first half

of this century.

Too Many Complaints

After ten months of sickness
she's complained about me
complaining all the time
she says i'm a whinger
& i complain far too much
& far too often

when i was first diagnosed
with cancer
she was at my bedside
daily often with flowers
& clean pyjamas
& she listened to me
complain

but that first night i came
home from hospital
she certainly didn't whinge
or complain
for two & a half hours
we were both dripping wet

& while i was complaining
fairly frequently throughout
my chemo & radio when i was
back in hospital
she wasn't complaining

especially after i got her onto
my bed in the private room

lately though—
she has been complaining
in fact she's gone on for weeks
how come you haven't
written a poem about me for
five years?
how come you haven't
got beer in the fridge for me
like you used to?
how come you never
come to my place & i always
have to come to yours?
how come you are always
grumpy?

last Saturday night she
repeated her new line
i'm too tired

frankly so am i.

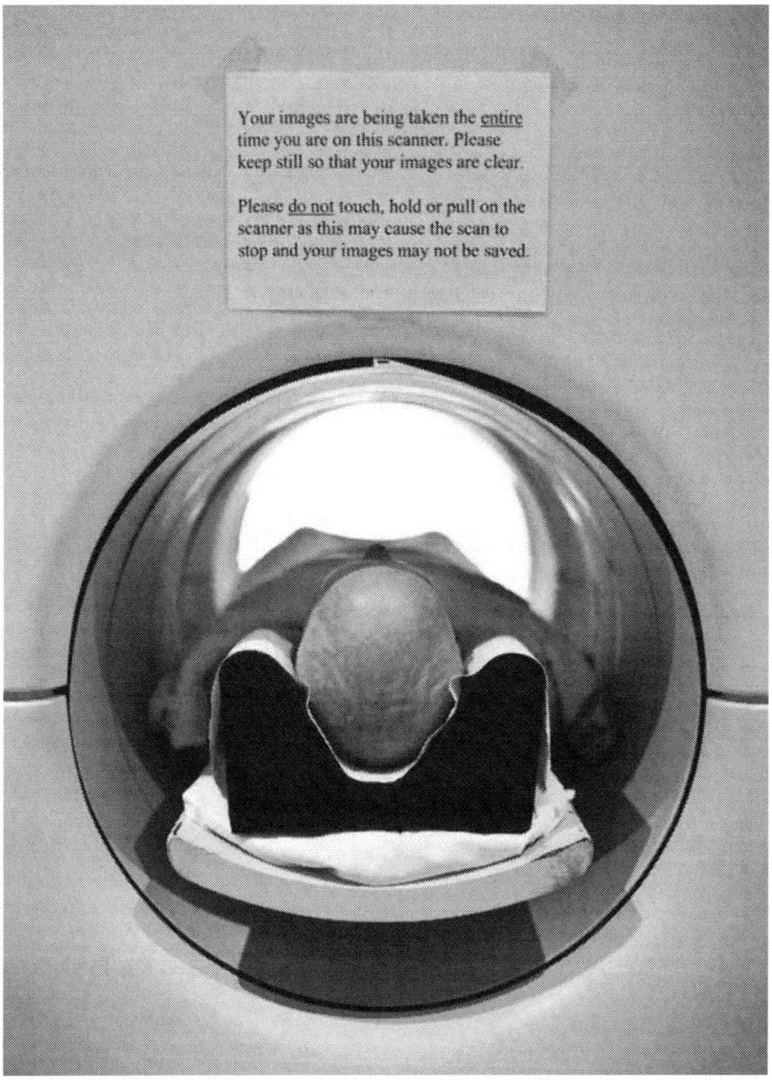
Your images are being taken the entire time you are on this scanner. Please keep still so that your images are clear.
Please do not touch, hold or pull on the scanner as this may cause the scan to stop and your images may not be saved.

Reversing

I was reversing out of my driveway
& signalled to a bloke
to move his car which was in my way

he was a young man twenty—
maybe twenty-two lots of bottle
blond hair tousled & spiky
& his car was about as old
as him

he was parked in a **No Parking** zone
& it pissed me off
as i turned out i drew alongside him—
rolled down my window & growled
can't you read you idiot it says
no parking

he looked at me momentarily & said
chill out dude

i set the car into drive
took a left turn slowly—
& drove down the road laughing

he was right
of course.

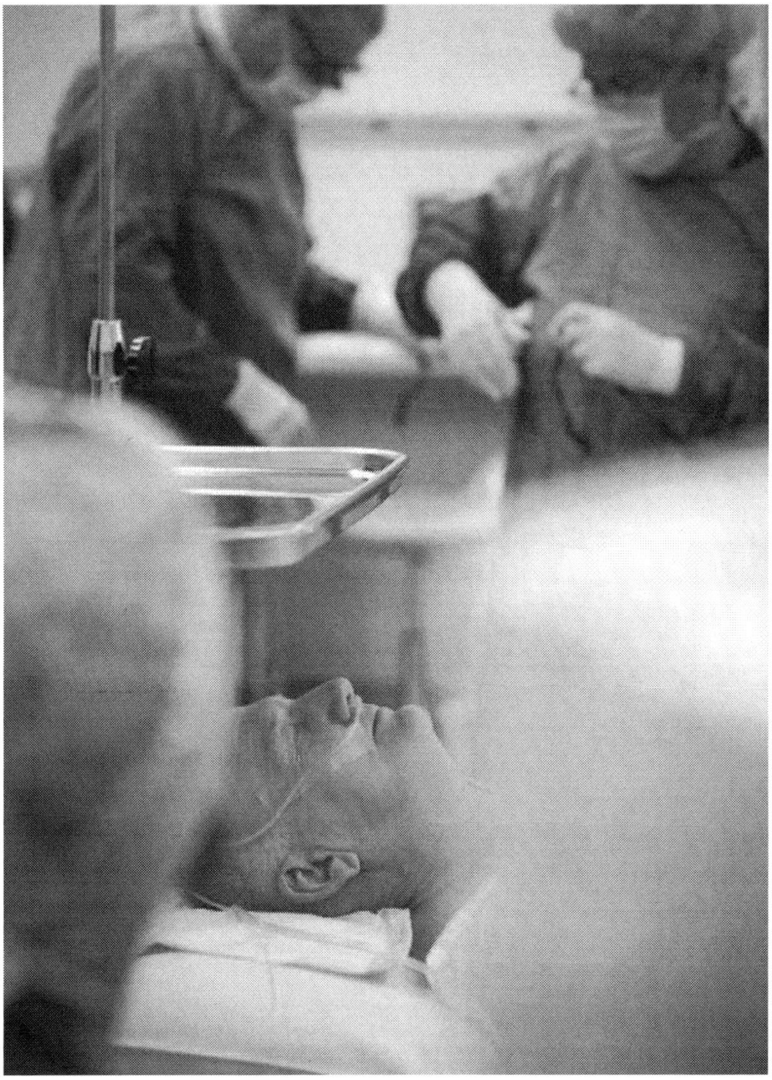

The Day I Dropped Several e's

For the best part of five
months
i'd been rendered
almost voiceless

i'd adopted the nickname
'Whispering Geoff'
along with a habit of ringing
a small brass bell
to get my daughter's attention

& when out shopping in my
neighbourhood
i could no longer yell across
the broad road to a passing friend
& i was far too weak
to pick up pace

so when the surgeon suggested
an implant to replace
the voice box on my left side
i was more than keen

he suggested it would be like
a piece of coral

with holes running through it
both ways
& it would bounce the sounds
made from my right side
so they'd amplify

on the day of the op i was
given a white gown
a pair of white stockings—
then shown to a cubicle

i was told to leave my underpants on

i don't normally wear stockings
& when i rolled them on & looked
into the mirror i thought
maybe black fishnets
would look better with my red jocks
but i remained mute

in the theatre i was given an
understanding of the protocol
& then a full anaesthetic

i was told that mid-way through
the procedure i was to be roused
& asked to speak
the insert was then to be moved
around to achieve my natural voice

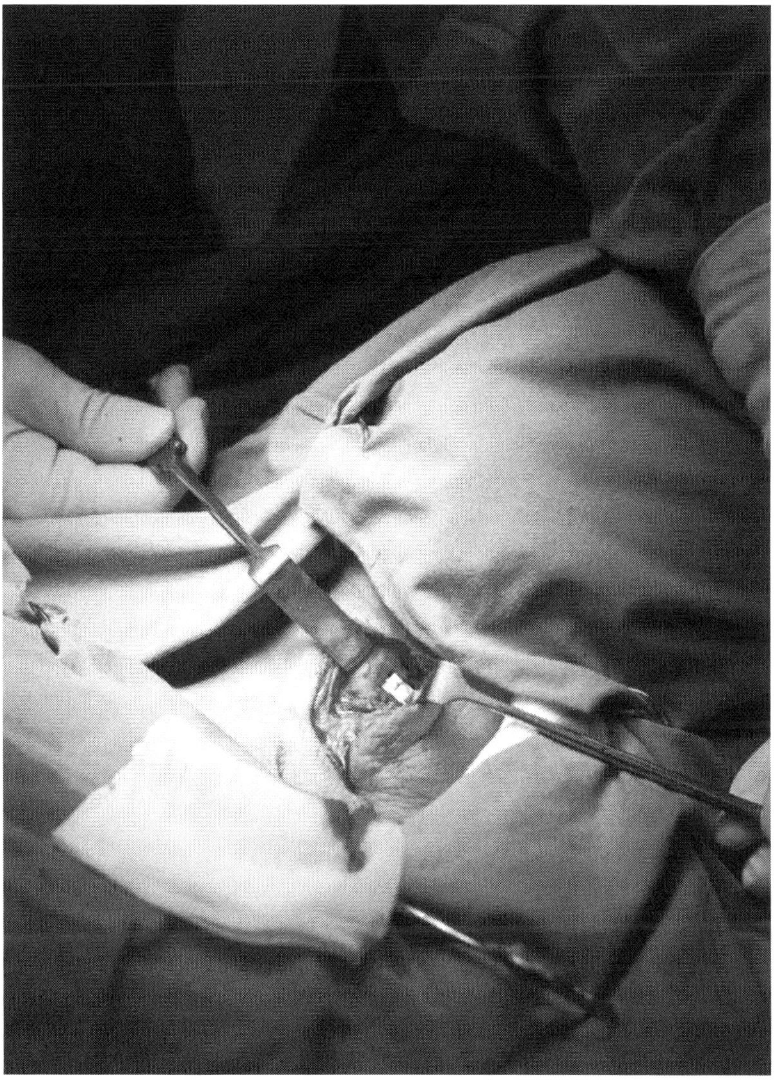

before i was sent off i said
you'd better not put in a Chinese
insert i want to be able to speak
normally when i wake up

when i was brought around i remember
feeling quite clear
the surgeon said

in a moment i'm going to insert
the prosthesis & tune it to suit
your natural voice
i'd like you then to say 'e'
for me several times

i told him i'd like to see the
prosthesis first

we can't do that if i drop it
the operation will have to cease
we can't play games...
i want you to be a good boy
& do what you are told

say 'e' for me now
that's good very good
now keep repeating 'e'
until i tell you to stop

after several soundings he said
that's enough
we're going to put you back
to sleep now
we'll talk soon

about thirty minutes later
we did.

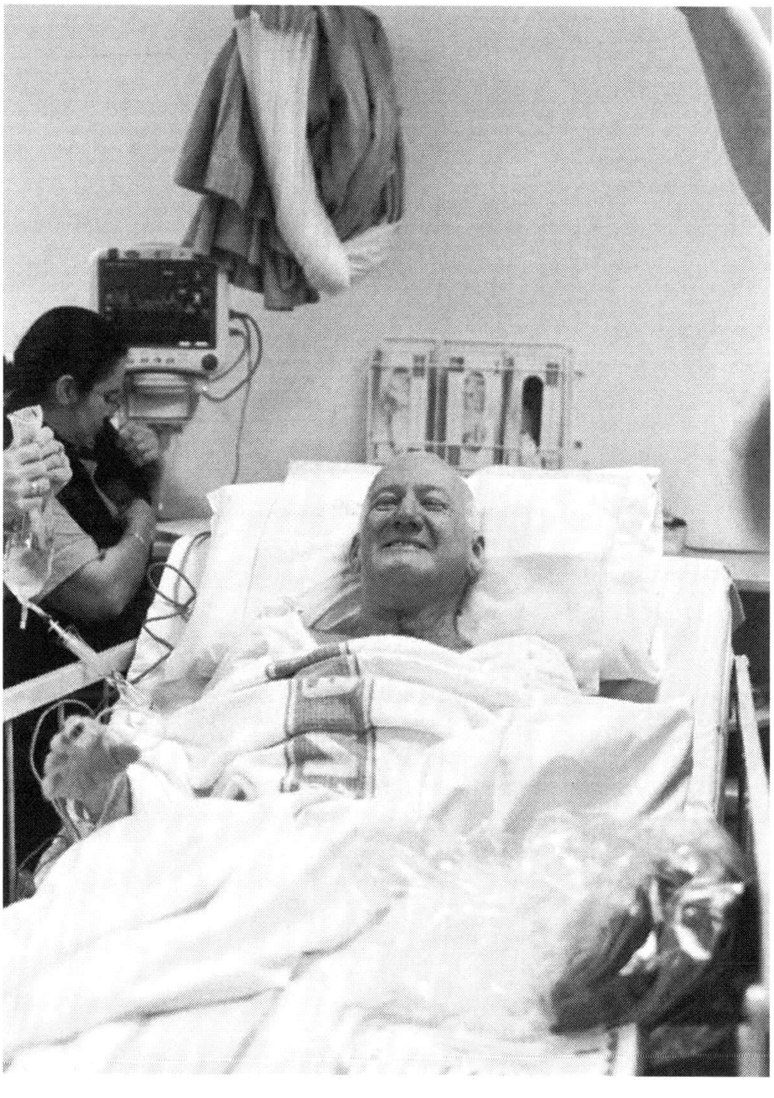

An Uncertain Future

I was sitting in my car opposite
the Adelaide Magistrates Court
waiting on a change of lights
when i first saw her

she was in her early twenties
had on a black sleeveless top
& a denim mini skirt
her arms & legs were heavily
tanned & she wore strappy sandals

her hair was bottle blonde—
& as she crossed in front of me
blowing out a stream of blue
cigarette smoke
i noticed her black roots
complemented her chipped & broken
front teeth

she was at least seven months pregnant

the lights changed
i moved off slowly—
into my own uncertain future.

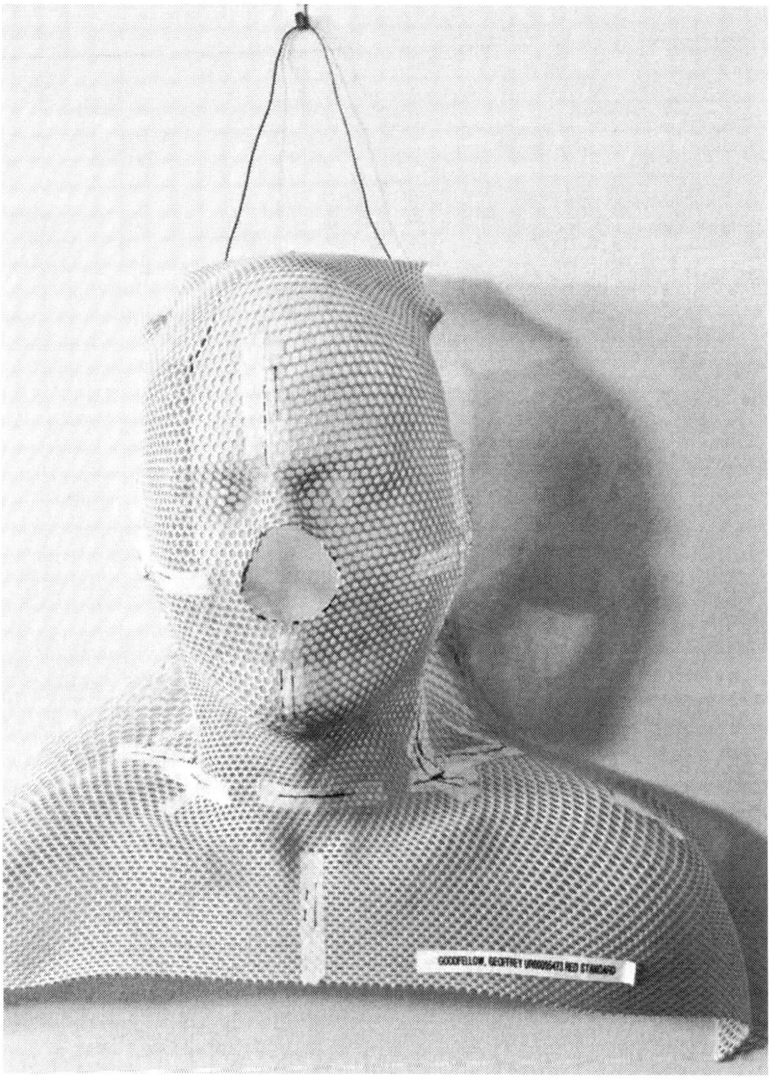
GOODFELLOW, GEOFFREY
RED STANDARD

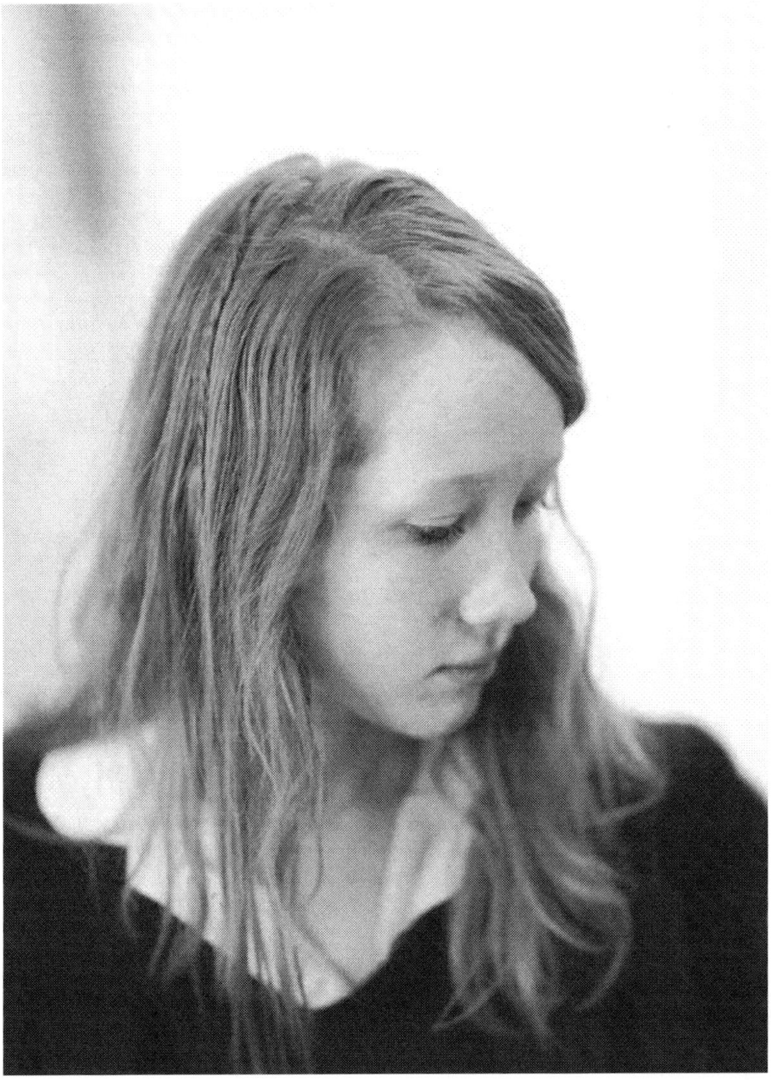

the c word

Story by
Grace Goodfellow

For my Pappa Bear–
Obviously

And also for Elli–
Sadness is the ocean and you are teaching me how to swim.

I adore you both.

Prologue

Once upon a time, when the birds chewed lime, and the monkeys chewed tobacco – he was okay.

He taught me how to read, and how to write, and how to play hopscotch. He showed me how to throw a frisbee properly, how to bake scones and the best way to tie your shoelaces. (And also how to break a stained-glass window, with said frisbee.) He played a game with me; maybe a hundred times. It was supposed to teach me about alliteration (and improve my hand-eye co-ordination skills). I laughed because I loved hearing him announce, *And next up, we've got Ingriiiid ... the Idiot!*

He read me nursery rhymes, and used different accents for each one. He bought me an icy pole every day after school, and he let me sit on his shoulders; so I could see the world.

From up there, high on his sunburnt shoulders, it was beautiful.

Everything was perfect.

And all of a sudden, Friday became the most significant day of the week

The very first Friday was my very first day of year eleven. There I was, in my new school dress, standing in the middle of the mall. It'd been a tiring and confusing and headache-inducing week – and I was glad to be amongst friends. We stood around, telling stories and laughing and generally being obnoxious.

Bella was there, and every now and then she'd glance at me. I remember her asking, 'So he's home then?' and I remember her smile when I nodded. We talked about our new stationery and all the homework we'd been given and how sad it was about Heath Ledger. We giggled when the Saint Peter's boys sauntered past and sighed about the weather.

Nothing really happened. It was a normal Friday afternoon. This is what we always did. We stood around and we talked and we laughed and we yelled out silly things to our friends who happened to walk past. I met Kyle, a shy boy with skin the colour of coffee. He inquired as to how I'd found the first week of year eleven. I shrugged my shoulders and said, 'It was okay. My dad's been a bit sick, so I've been a little stressed. But it's all right.' He smiled gently, but did not ask further questions.

And then my phone rang.

This was not an unusual occurrence. Dad would usually ring to ask what train I'd be on, or to tell me, *Come home soon, please.* This time, there was no warning sign. Nothing. It was just like every other time.

'Where are you, my darling daughter?'

'In Rundle Mall, with Bel and the twins and some other Pulteney people. Ms Simpson found me today and told me you were home. So I thought I'd celebrate.'

'Well, when's the next train? She must have got the message wrong, because I told her to tell you to come home.'

'Ah, she's so silly. I'll be on the 5.07, okay?'

'No worries. I'll see you then.'

And that was it.

Just like every other time.

I said goodbye to my friends, promising that we'd catch up soon. I remember them all waving madly and carrying on. Alex was laughing, and his eyes were dancing. I remember thinking, *This year, I will kiss him.* I thought a lot of things about year eleven, actually. Things like:

- how my biology teacher was really annoying
- how I would miss Hungry Jacks on Fridays
- how much homework I would have and
- how stupid it was choosing design.

I thought: *This year – this year will be beautiful.*

And I believed it.

Dishes and Daddy's lap

He was fine in the car. Happy, even. He and my brother cracked jokes about the 'hot boys in Rundle Mall' and Paul added – 'Like, oh my god.

Those Saint Peter's guys are like, *soooo* hot.' I played along, joining in the laughter.

I asked Dad how he was, and he smiled gently. I took that as a 'Not bad, thanks' which was his standard response.

As we pulled into the driveway, I noticed Fiona standing at the kitchen window. She appeared to be washing the dishes, and I smiled. 'Lucky someone's doing them, hey,' I said. Dad and Paul nodded.

It was such an ordinary day.

Well, not really. My sister-in-law never usually did our dishes, but apart from that ... completely and utterly ordinary.

Inside, it was cool and quiet. Fiona embraced me, and I noticed a redness to her eyes. She was overly chatty; manic almost. And that's when I stopped. Dad was sitting at the kitchen table, across from Paul. They both looked at me. And I saw guilt on their faces.

Guilt and fear and hurt and worry.

Dad slapped his thigh three times. I walked over slowly, and sat down.

And that's when I knew, my year would not be beautiful.

The Truth

This is what he said: 'Gracie girl ... I'm really sorry. I wasn't honest with you the other day. I wanted to protect you, until I knew. The lump isn't just an infected abscess.

It's cancer.

And I'm so sorry. I wanted to tell you. But I was scared. And I knew you would be, too. They told me I've got up to five years. And I told them to get fucked, because I've got a sixteen-year-old daughter, and that I *have* to be at her twenty-first. I'm going to fight this. I will. I'll fight it. I won't leave you. I promise. I'm not going to let it get me. I'm not. Don't cry, darling. Shhh ... don't cry. It'll be okay. It will.'

And this is what I remember thinking:

He's going to die.

So then what happened, was this

We cried and talked and discussed the options. We paused and reflected and we wiped our eyes and we sniffed and we looked at each other.

We cried some more. We hugged and sighed and we thought, *Fuck. This can't be happening.* We sobbed and we let the grief take over, momentarily. We gave in to the sadness and hugeness of it all. And then I changed out of my school uniform and I looked in the mirror, and I said out loud: 'I am the girl with the dad who has cancer.'

We rang our closest friends and our favourite family members. We cried and laughed and told Dad to stop making stupid jokes. There was an underlying sadness. I am not denying that. But as the evening progressed, there was also a little bit of hope. And a little bit of optimism. And a little bit of 'oh, you're such a pain in the neck!'.

I rang my friends in alphabetical order. And I told them. Many promised to look after me. Others promised sleepovers and late night phone calls.

Almost everyone promised me he would be okay.

We sat around all night; me and Dad and Paul and Fiona and various other family members. We told stories and we laughed at Dad's hospital jokes and we ate and we drank and we carried on. We did what we do best. We bullshitted our way through it. Everyone was terrified but we still laughed. And all of a sudden, the first Friday was over. The journey had begun, but at least that particular day had ended.

Tell me about the Seven Stages of Grief

Shock and Denial?

Yeah, there was a bit of that. A lot of people found it hard to believe. I was numb to it, for a while. I remember thinking, *He can't die. He can't. I want him to be okay.*

Our friends, the ones in Semaphore – they thought we were lying. Jackie's response to the news was 'Bullshit!' We shook our heads.

And then she cried.

It became a fact; you know, like, how you tell people you're a Virgo or whatever. Or that you're a vegetarian. We went into shops and homes and banks. And the phrase 'I have cancer' became just like the revelation of your star sign. It didn't lose its meaning. It just ... became an easier thing to say.

What about Pain and Guilt?

Yep, that too. I remember lying in bed, sobbing uncontrollably. It hurt. *I* felt sick. I didn't try and escape it. I didn't drink or go out partying or take drugs. I didn't hurt myself. I just cried, a lot.

I felt guilty, too. Because sometimes I was just so *angry* with him, and so terrified about the possibility of losing him – that I lashed out. I remember thinking, *I shouldn't have to look after him. But I am. Because I love him, and because I want him to get better. But right now,* he's *making* me *feel sick.*

I felt guilty about never doing the dishes. About not hanging the clothes on the line. About rolling my eyes when he said something. About name calling and yelling and disagreeing. About wishing he'd just *SHUT UP.*

And how about Anger and Bargaining?

I didn't blame anyone. I couldn't. But I did ask why a lot. I did cry a lot. I did think a lot. And I used to pray, too. I used to pray that I'd get a boyfriend, or a gig at the Governor Hindmarsh. But now I started praying for Dad.

I'll be good. I'll be a really, really good person if you just make him better.

Did you feel Depressed, or Lonely? And how about Reflecting – did you do any of that?

I felt depressed sometimes. But not lonely. I surrounded myself with people. Friends helped me 'forget' – or at least to take the edge off it all. I didn't know how to deal with it. How are you ever supposed to know?

I felt despair, yes. And a little bit empty. But mostly, I just felt scared.

The encouragement from others, you know, it was helpful. But I preferred them to be realistic. And it was hard to really know what was going to happen. So, most of the time, we'd just ... be silent.

And then there's the Upward Turn – do you want to tell me about that?

Yeah. I guess I began to adjust to the idea. Things became a little calmer, at least before the surgery and treatment. I stopped feeling sick and just focused on getting through it all with him. I remembered all the stuff he said, about fighting it.

And I started to believe him.

And then what?

We started talking about surgery and chemo and radiation. We waited for the hospital to contact us. We were still sad, but we began to seek realistic solutions. We worked through it, step by step.

Right, and then you began to accept it? Did you feel a sense of Hope?

Yeah, totally. I accepted it, and dealt with the reality of the situation. I met the surgeon and I googled 'throat cancer' and I cried and laughed and dreamt and thought. I wasn't happy necessarily, but I began to see that, eventually, it would all be beautiful again.

Just keep the noise down, okay?

My closest friends, who I referred to fondly as 'The Pond' came over one night in February. We sat in the lounge room and we laughed. We laughed a lot, actually. It was exactly what I needed, and I think it made Dad happy too. Especially since we were relatively quiet and well-behaved.

No one really asked how he was going. But that was okay. I didn't even *want* to talk about cancer or treatment or tears. I wanted to talk about the up-coming formals and drinking and how rat's tails are disgusting and beer and what we'd all do once school was over. We took silly photos and sat in the back yard and Kyle held onto me – and for just a moment, I felt safe.

We reminisced and we giggled and we swore and carried on. We made promises. We hugged and Bella played my guitar.

It was perfect.

No.

It was beautiful.

Good Friday

He went into surgery, and I went to Kangaroo Island. By then, I was sort of ... *used* to the idea. Well, as much as you can be.

I went away with my mum and our family friends, as well as a close childhood friend. We spent days on the beach taking silly photos. We ate Easter eggs and taught two-year-old Noah to say duck. We told stories and stayed up late. We watched movies and got sunburnt and wore flannies. We played board games and we giggled and we never spoke about Dad.

He rang me, though. His voice had changed dramatically. It was a shock, I guess, even though we'd been warned. Some of the tumour had been welded to his voice box and there was nerve damage. He sounded ... old, and sick. Which I guess he was. I can't remember what I thought, or how I felt. I guess relieved. I knew that the surgery was a walk in the park compared to the six weeks of radiation ahead of him. But I also knew that he *would* fight.

He'd promised.

And then, it all just sort of ... kept on keeping on

A lot of things happened. Kyle became my boyfriend. Dad became 'Scarface' (care of my friend

Chelsea). I became somewhat content with the whole shenanigans. I went to a music festival, Dad went into hospital – you know, the usual.

And then more stuff happened. I broke up with Kyle. Dad became 'Whispering Geoff' (care of himself). I became somewhat frightened by the whole shenanigans.

By this time, it was May. Dad had begun chemo and I had begun sleeping in seventeen hour blocks. I put it down to exhaustion, stress, blah blah blah. I went to my year eleven formal, and I felt ... free. Just for a little while, I didn't have to worry about Dad and whether or not he had a headache, or if his neck was red. I was allowed to be a sixteen-year-old girl, in a pretty blue dress, with a handsome young man on her arm. I was still 'the girl whose dad has cancer', but it was my subheading, you know? People still asked. At the afterparty, friends from other schools and girls I'd never really spoken to before approached me. Gently they asked, 'And how's your dad going? Is he okay?'

I nodded, a lot of the time. And I fought back tears when a school friend, whose mother had died from cancer when we were in year seven, held my hand and told me that it would be okay. She said, '*It* will be okay, *he* will be okay, and *you* will be okay.'

And then I cried.

Remember Love

I'd been writing CD reviews for *Rip It Up* magazine, and had stumbled across a musician by the name of Michael Peter. This singer-songwriter from the Central Coast not only provided me with beautiful music but Dad with a 'theme song' for the year. Dad and I often listened to CDs in the car and we had always shared a similar taste in music. Despite his inability to sing – or to understand the concept of a melody – he really did have a good appreciation for music. The final track on Michael's *Patched Up Heart* EP – entitled 'Remember Love' – became a kind of anthem for my dad. Lines like 'Cheer up, boy, don't let it get you down' really resonated with him. If the CD was in the car he always requested that particular track.

And then, in early May, Dad was able to request the song – but this time, in person. Michael had begun playing 'Invade the lounge room' gigs, which sounds a lot less suss then you'd imagine. Apparently, playing in people's lounge rooms was a favourite way for Michael to perform. After a bowl of pumpkin soup and a quick round of introductions, we headed upstairs. One of the 'audience' members asked, 'So, got any good stories, Michael?'

His answer? 'I do indeed. *Plenty* of good stories.' And with that, he began to play.

I remember thinking, *This is ... magic. Here is this young musician sitting in my lounge room playing absolutely beautiful music.* As he sang, a smile crept onto his face, as well as everyone else's in the room.

Especially Dad's.

Everything about Michael, his music, his smile, was so relaxed and so honest.

As the night progressed, stories were told, jokes were shared and some truly amazing songs were performed. Dad tried his best to sing along with 'Remember Love' – and Michael was touched by the revelation of it being the Goodfellow's 'anthem' for 2008.

We were cheered up immensely.

And, we had a new friend.

'You look like an elephant'

A few weeks after Michael's visit, Dad had the naso-gastric tube inserted. Cue stupid jokes about it being a phone, him looking like an elephant and ... well, they didn't get much funnier than that.

His then-girlfriend Emily referred to the tins of Ensure as sounding like a feminine hygiene product. Instead, they were cans of something-flavoured drinks. Dad would syringe the liquid up into the tube. It was the only thing he could consume, much to his disgust.

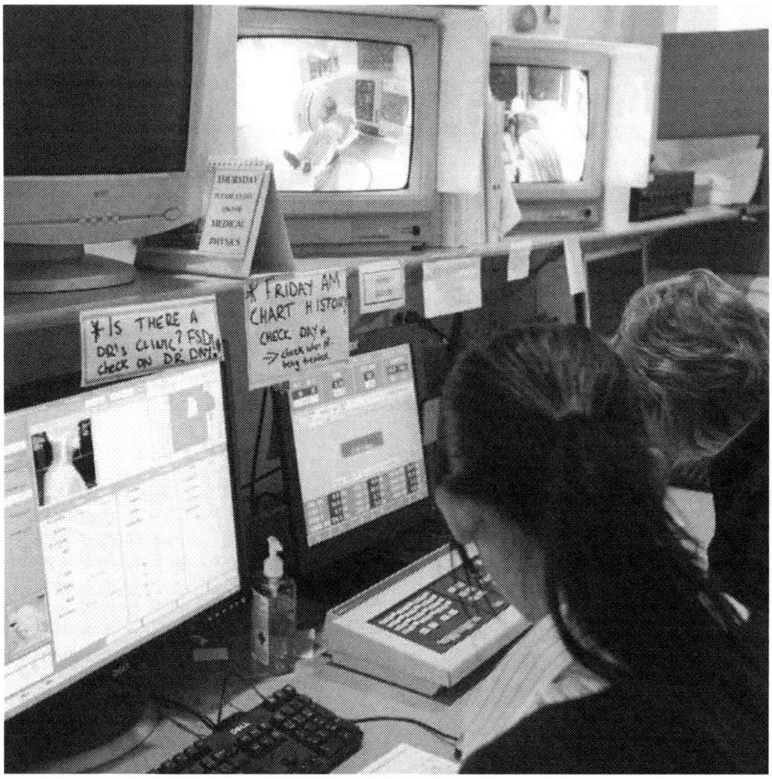

The radiation was getting to him. Five days a week he would be driven, by my ever-lovely brother Paul, into the city. The Oncology Ward became his second home. I visited once, just to suss it out. It was strange – seeing my dad on this huge spaceship-looking machine. From the room, we could watch the procedure on a little black and white television. The radiation nurses tried to explain what was going on, but I took little of it in. I remember thinking, *This is* so *weird.* And I remember when Dad emerged from the room, unclipped and unmasked, his look of ... relief, I think it was. Like he was glad it was over. At least for another day.

The feeding tube remained, and the nausea appeared. His neck became a crusty, red mess. He spent hours crying and retching and 'having a lie down'. Eventually, it became so *bad* he was readmitted to hospital. This was a *bad* time. I was due to travel to Orange in NSW to spend time with friends. I was reluctant to go, but also glad to get away from the dramas.

Things were not looking beautiful, at all.

O-Town

I went to Orange, against my better judgement. The first night I was there a whole group of family friends visited me at my cousin's house. I was tired and worried and a little bit flat. Sam, the boy I have been in love with since I was nine years old, was there. And even he couldn't cheer me up. I was standing in the kitchen. He was on the other side, looking at me intently. 'How's your dad, Grace?'

I wanted to cry; to reach out and have him hold me. I remember thinking, *I don't want to tell you. Because then I will collapse.*

I remembered the previous night. Dad had come over to my mum's house. He'd cried, a lot. And he'd told me that he wanted to just 'go away'. I remember the despair I felt. I scribbled frantically in my diary, writing *'And I keep saying maybe he's just in denial ... but what if he isn't? What if he's dying?'*

I remember thinking, *I hate EVERYTHING. He's MEANT to be okay. He said he'd fight this.* And I remember the look on Sam's face when I said, 'Not very good.'

The trip, however, was good. Despite an upsetting phone call to Dad on the first night, the rest of my visit was beautiful. I went to one of Sam's friend's houses, and we drank beer and laughed and talked about how it'd been snowing. I held Sam's hand and I sat on the roof of his mate's car and looked up at the stars. I didn't talk about what was happening back in Adelaide. I just focused on the good stuff.

Are You Old Enough

And then there was the benefit gig. Dad's Irish mate Con had organised it all. Lots of singers and creative people were there. And our friends. Hundreds of them. I sang with my friends Luke and Elli. The set list was a surprise, and much to Dad's delight we played his favourite song, 'Are You Old Enough'. Years ago, in the car, the song had been playing. Well, a cover of it. Dad told me how it was his favourite and we laughed about the ... *relevance* ... of some of the lyrics. I had asked him, 'I know it won't be for a long time but ... can we play this song at your funeral?'

He laughed, and said, 'Good idea.' Little did I know that only three years later I would be performing it at a benefit concert designed to raise money to support him during his battle with cancer.

The night was lovely; lots of singing and speeches and smiles. Dad was dressed in his best suit, and the naso-gastric tube was nowhere to be seen. He looked *brilliant.* Which, you know, was a surprise considering three weeks earlier he had basically given up.

We danced together and we hugged and we saw that, maybe, maybe this wasn't such a terrible year after all.

Lately, things have been changing

He stopped drinking coffee and started wearing socks to bed. He ate slowly, spoke quietly, and wept less. A lot of the time, I felt ... frustrated. Because I couldn't fix him or help him or make it better.

But I tried.

I *let* him wear his slippers without teasing him.

And I *let* him whinge.

And I *let* him make annoying noises as he ate.

And I *let* him swear profusely, without telling him to stop.

And I *let* him hate this whole thing. Because I hated it, too.

Happy Birthday, to you

The day before I turned seventeen he went back into hospital. This time for something less serious. They were going to put a prosthetic vocal cord in so his voice could return to 'normal'. I went into the

Royal Adelaide after school and found him sitting up in bed. He smiled wildly and said, 'Happy birthday, Gracie.'

And I burst into tears, because he sounded like my daddy again. It was the best birthday present ever.

Agggghhhh!!!

By mid September, he was on the mend. His voice was a little stronger. So, that gave him permission to yell at me. Which he did a lot.

I had all these hideous fights with him. And I remember thinking, *He hates me.*

Of course, he didn't. And of course, we got over it. I think, it was just ... overwhelming. He was grumpy and tired and sore and his *tongue hurt,* and didn't I get sick of hearing that?!

I didn't, or couldn't understand why he was being such a drama queen. No, that's not true. I understood, but I felt as if he didn't care that *I* was suffering, too. The seventeen hour sleeps became more frequent; my muscles ached, I couldn't concentrate, I was lethargic and bored and fed up with hearing about how his mouth had been burnt. He didn't realise that it had affected me.

Or maybe he did. We never really talked about it.

Things That Can Give You Cancer

Coke

Listerine
Burnt toast
Microwaves
Smoking
Drinking alcohol
Passive smoking
Drugs
Foundation
Roll-on deodorant
Aerosol cans
Too much sunshine
Not enough sunshine
Paint thinners
Mobile phones
Solariums
Leaving detergent suds on your dishes
Processing photos
Drinking tea that is too hot

No, really, I wasn't kidding about the Friday thing

And then things started to calm down. Once again, I found myself in Rundle Mall with a group of friends. There were people *everywhere* and the sun, ironically enough, was shining. Brittany and I were walking to Sportsgirl; the others had split off and were trying their luck in Myer. My phone beeped and when I saw 'Dad' on the screen, my heart began to race.

The message went a little like this: 'Got the all clear!' And once again, I found myself in tears. But this time, on this particular Friday; they were tears of joy. Tears of relief and happiness and hope and utter joy. They were beautiful tears, if that is possible.

I remember ringing him and just screaming. I didn't care if people pulled faces at me, or if they rolled their eyes. He was okay, and, as clichéd as it sounds – that is all that mattered.

In that moment his survival and *okay* S3 eliminated all other fears. Nothing else mattered.

We'd been sitting, waiting, wishing

We'd waited eight months for this.

Eight, long, tiresome months.

Eight months involving tears and hurt and misunderstandings.

Eight months of worry and regret and fear and laughter and fighting and wishing and praying and radiation and neck jokes and googling stuff and hugs and tantrums and hospitals.

Eight months of ... emotions that don't even have names yet.

Let's go

And then there was the Recuperation Tour. We drove to Melbourne, and I remember laughing a lot.

I remember, 'Put that ... aeroplane song on, Grace. That one's my favourite.'

I remember buying ice-cream after ice-cream, because his tongue still hurt.

I remember laughing and joking and, 'Yeah, this one's got a really nice melody.'

'Dad, do you even *know* what a melody *is?*'

And I remember, 'No. But I like saying it.'

Melbourne was great. We saw friends and we ate and got lost in St Kilda (*three* times). We had brunch at Mario's, one of our favourite restaurants. The waiter asked if we'd like some water. Dad said, 'Yeah, thanks,' and at the same time I shook my head. He stopped for a minute and said, 'Do you want one? Because if you do, you'd better tell me. There's a drought on, you know.'

For the rest of the trip, any time someone mentioned water, Dad would ask me to tell that story. It was nice, in a way, to have a father with a sense of humour again. He was back to normal, more or less. And that was the best thing ever.

Moo

Well, okay. Maybe not the *best thing ever.* But it was close.

The best thing ever was actually being on the farm. Not *our* farm, although it may as well be. Dad had known Bruce Roberts for over thirty years. They were good mates, and his family had become part of ours. Their dairy farm on the north-west coast of Tasmania had always been a place of solace. And now it was a place of rest. A place of recovering and relaxing and maybe a little bit of teasing (especially about the slippers).

I remember thinking, *It's peaceful here. And it feels like home.*

It was the perfect place for him to be. No, the perfect place for *us* to be.

Dad got out on the quad bikes and cooked up a storm for the four (or sometimes five) hungry farmers. We told stories and carried on and agreed with Jo when she said, 'Oh, it's just such a *bloody* relief!'

I spent a lot of time with Ollie, Bruce's eldest son. I'd always had a soft spot for him and it was nice to sit down and tell him about the year, and how I'd been feeling. It was nice, too, just being able to smile and laugh and joke about it. He cared, I knew that he cared – but I didn't feel as though it was necessary to make a big deal of it all. I was happy to talk about the introduction of socks in bed, and porridge in the morning. And I was happy to sigh occasionally and say, almost light-heartedly, 'Yeah, it was a shit year.' Because it was; it *had* been. And I felt comfortable enough to tell Ollie that I'd been angry a lot of the time. I felt comfortable enough to say, 'It was the worst year of my life.'

Dad and Bruce spent hours talking as well. Well, as much as they could considering Brucey was out tending to the cows a lot of the time. It was calving season and so they were all a little bit busy. It was nice in the evenings too. Sitting in front of the fire with farm dogs, Hash and Taco, at our feet. It was nice drinking hot chocolate and listening to eighteen-year-old Barnaby tell me: 'Only put it in for a minute ... *aaaaand* ... twenty seconds.' It was nice to sit with Ollie and laugh about how I still wasn't driving. It was nice to see Bruce relaxed and ever-attentive to Dad's possible needs or wants. In the past, Bruce and Dad had spent a lot of time teasing one another and carrying on. Bruce's dry sense of humour was still present, however he was ... gentle with Dad. It interested me to see how people's behaviour toward him changed. Jo was more or less the same – pointing out that we were all 'sick of hearing about the bloody cancer!'. And Ollie just wanted to know if he could still eat lamb shanks.

I felt grateful. Grateful for the freedom and the openness (not only of the land, but also of the conversation). I didn't want to go home. I just wanted to lay down in one of the paddocks and soak up the sunshine. I wanted to just ... be.

That's a big dam

We rode the quad bikes out to the newly installed dam. I sat on the back of Emily's bike and Dad led the expedition. He was in his element, although he looked slightly out of place in his jeans and baby blue hoodie. But he was smiling, and he had the air of someone who was feeling pretty great about life.

We stopped and admired the giant expanse of water. And then Dad attempted to put the bike into reverse. Let's just say he came *quite* close to ending up in said giant expanse of water.

The three of us laughed the whole way back to the farmhouse. And the laughter continued when I pulled out my camera, which I had (luckily) brought along for the ride. Ollie and Barnaby found it all very amusing, especially the part when Dad edged even closer to the dam. It was ... ironic, almost. Thinking, *He beat cancer, and yet he nearly drove a bright red quad bike into a dam this afternoon.*

Silly thing.

I'm so sleeeeeeepy

Life returned to normal. Well, there was a greater sense of normality at least.

Dad still found eating difficult – but found solace and comfort in chocolate custard.

I went back to school. This was in no way enjoyable. I was devastatingly tired, just totally exhausted. It was strange – because all of a sudden I became the 'sick' one. I missed a lot of school opting for hours and hours of uninterrupted sleep instead.

On Friday 31st (see, I *told* you) we drove to the doctor's surgery. I'd been there not even a week earlier when I had been told I was suffering from a relapse of glandular fever. I'd had a blood test, and was 'eagerly' awaiting the results. We sat in the waiting room and I said to Dad, 'So if they're okay, can I go to Karley's tonight?' I was looking forward to the Halloween party, even though I didn't have a costume planned. I think I was more looking forward to getting out of the house, actually. Having been bedridden for a week, I was longing for the outside world.

I sat in the chair, across from the doctor. He smiled gently and I recognised it instantly. It was a 'wow, I feel sorry for you' smile.

I began to think: *What if I have cancer too you can't catch it I know that but still it would explain why I've been so tired and sore and I've heard you can get tumours from stress and I HAVE been pretty stressed lately oh shit what if it's chronic fatigue what if I never get better I really don't want to do year thirteen but I might have to why are my legs SO SORE this is ridiculous all I want to do is sleep and not wake up.*

And then Dr Alex Alexander (yes, that was his name) said quietly, 'Now, we have received the results of your blood tests. Your white blood cell count is very low and, obviously, the Epstein-Barr virus is present. Usually, when you relapse from glandular fever more than three times, we call it chronic fatigue syndrome. Have you heard of this before?' I nodded slowly. Tears began to well in my eyes.

He spoke to me about resting and drinking plenty of fluids and gentle exercise. I was numb; totally and utterly numb. I remember walking back to the waiting room, tears streaking my face. I pressed my hand against the wall, so as to steady myself. I remember the look of worry on Dad's face as Dr Alexander explained what was going on. I remember being embraced by my dad and asking, in between sobs, 'This means I can't go to Karley's tonight, doesn't it?'

I cried the whole way home. I wrote my best friend Annie a text message, telling her. I remember closing my eyes and saying, 'I just want to go to sleep.'

I remember the look of guilt on Dad's face. I think he partly blamed himself. Of course, it wasn't his fault but I could tell he felt somewhat responsible. And maybe, you know, the stress of the whole cancer thing had had an impact – but I was hardly going to hold him responsible for a lifetime condition. I couldn't blame my aching legs or my inability to concentrate on my dad. Just like his diagnosis, mine was unfair.

I slept a lot and cried a lot and messaged my friends a lot. I lay in bed and looked at the ceiling. I sighed deeply and wished it all away.

The first few days were awful. I gave in to the illness because I didn't have the strength or want to fight it. I let the fatigue and pain take over. I didn't miss my friends, I didn't miss going to school, I didn't miss having to wake up at seven o'clock in the morning to catch the train. I didn't care about anything. I just wanted to sleep.

Ouch

And that's exactly what I did. When I wasn't sleeping I was crying.

And when I wasn't crying – well, you can fill in the gaps.

I remember one particular afternoon, I was, not surprisingly, in bed. My legs were aching and I was so tired it hurt. I remember yelling out for Dad, but my bedroom door was closed and he was lying down in his room with Emily. I couldn't move. Hot tears ran down my face as I screamed out for him. I sobbed. It was maybe five or ten minutes until he came into my bedroom looking flustered and utterly concerned.

'What's wrong, Gracie?'

Emily was at his side, and she looked equally worried.

'My ... legs ... hurt.'

'Let's get you into the shower, Gracie. That'll make you feel better.'

I shook my head, with the little energy I had. 'I can't ... move.' Emily looked at me lovingly and said, 'We'll carry you, and put a chair in the shower.'

I lifted myself up, slowly and surely, and when my feet hit the carpet I cried out in pain. Dad returned to his room to grab a chair, and Emily helped me walk across the hallway to the bathroom. I couldn't stop crying. I sat on the closed lid of the toilet, undressing at the speed of a ninety-year-old woman. I sat on the red chair and cried because I felt pathetic.

I felt only slightly better once I was wrapped in my towel. I shuffled back to my bedroom and the tears began to flow again. Dad came in shortly after and sat on the edge of my bed.

'If I hadn't been sick, then you probably wouldn't be, either.'

Again, it was the guilt thing – but still, I couldn't hold him responsible. I shook my head and told him no, it was because I hadn't looked after myself properly. He accepted it, to a degree – saying it was a lot to do with stress, and he was unsure what he could do. All *I* could do was cry. I longed for days of running on the beach, doing somersaults and eight hours of sleep – as opposed to sixteen or seventeen.

My best friend Annie told me, 'I don't want you to have even the smallest slither of fatigue, let alone a chronic amount.'

I didn't either, but there was very little I could do about it. Other than the obvious.

Yes.

Sleep.

School and stuff

I started going to school again. Just in the mornings, until recess. It was hard; harder than I'd expected anyway. Of course the teachers were lovely and understanding and sympathetic. And, of course, I used it as an excuse for just about everything.

We used to sit in a big circle at recess and lunchtime. Upon my return to school I stopped sitting and started lying down. I stretched out on the cement, closed my eyes and imagined I was in my nice, comfy bed. Occasionally, one of the girls would throw something at me, just to make sure I was okay. It was a sign of affection and I was pleased to be back among friends.

My friendship with Elli and Luke had grown and developed since the benefit gig, and I'd started writing songs. Melbourne singer–songwriter Dom Cooley had seen some of the videos on YouTube and contacted me, asking whether we were keen to play with him at the Grace Emily Hotel the following month. I was stoked. Chelsea, a fellow muso, asked whether we'd like a 'special brass soloist'. Luke, Elli and I thought this a quite excellent idea and from there spent hours coming up with a name for our newly formed band.

Eventually, we decided on Darling Street. It felt ... *right* – and the rehearsal process began.

Otorhinolaryngology

Dad enforced an eight o'clock bedtime rule and I began studying for exams. My legs ached and my concentration levels fluctuated, but I still managed to have something of a life.

During the first week or so of November, Dad developed an infection. We weren't entirely sure what was wrong – but he didn't look well. He was headachy and lethargic and eventually found himself back in his second home – The Royal Adelaide Hospital.

I tried to carry on as normal, which was difficult, considering I was about to complete my end-of-year exams. Elli suggested I stay at her house, so that she could look after me. She promised to let me go to bed at eight o'clock and giggled when I told her she was an idiotface.

The heat was sweltering. We traipsed through the glass office doors and sighed as the November surprise heatwave hit us. Earlier I'd asked if she minded dropping into the hospital to check on Dad. She didn't, and so we made the long journey down North Terrace. I checked my phone to find the message containing the directions. He was in North Ward and Elli was amazed at my ability to find my way around.

Dad was quite cheery, relieved it was simply a blood infection easily managed by antibiotics and bed rest. He laughed at the two of us, carrying on and attempting to read the sign above his bed. I took a photo on my phone and dared Elli to pronounce the word.

'Otor – something – ology?' We laughed, and wondered aloud as to what exactly it was the study of.

We didn't stay long, but I think Dad was grateful for the visit and the hugs.

I know *I* was.

Can I see some ID, thanks?

Elli, Luke and I spent afternoons practising; sometimes in Allan's music store and sometimes in our backyards. We had mock arguments and re-wrote the set list over and over. The days and weeks just seemed to fly. Music and overdue assignments and the long-awaited warm weather all kind of just ... blurred together.

Our big moment arrived. It was hot, even at five in the afternoon. We'd agreed to meet at the Grace Em, just to run through a few things. I was buzzing, and couldn't wait to jump up on stage. I felt beautiful in my new blue dress and I was excited at the prospect of singing in front of a whole group of people. We sat inside, near the stage, and Luke tuned and re-tuned his guitar. We laughed nervously and wished aloud that we were eighteen – because it really *would* be nice to have a beer. Luke scoffed and said, 'Yeah, like I'm going to buy you girls a drink.' We rolled our eyes and laughed.

Even during the sound check I was smiling. It all seemed to be coming together, and I couldn't wait to look out into the crowd and say, 'This next song's for my dad.' I couldn't wait to play our newly revised version of 'Are You Old Enough' or to dance gracefully as we covered Angus and Julia's song 'Silver Coin'.

And I especially couldn't wait to sing my own song – 'Handstands'.

It was all so exciting, and this was heightened by the arrival of Dom. That feeling of excitement and awe lasted roughly ... five seconds. He was patronising and sarcastic but I smiled and said, 'Yeah, thanks heaps for this. We've been rehearsing all day.' He said, in a deadpan voice, 'Yeah, cool, well you kids should have fun.'

By six, we were sound-checked out, and decided to go on a search for dinner. We left the guitar, amp, shaker and trumpet sitting in a corner and stepped back out into the heat. On the way, we joked and laughed and carried on like the teenagers we were. The nerves had started to kick in, as well as a throbbing headache. Elli proceeded to crack 'muso/drug' jokes and the nerves subsided. I devoured pizza and Panadol and we took silly photos of one another. Dad messaged asking what time we were due to hit the stage, and I ran through the song lyrics in my head, wondering aloud about which of my friends would be sitting in front of the stage, hopefully singing along.

We headed back, and the butterflies took off again. As we made our way through the arch toward the stage, the blonde bartender stopped us in our tracks. She looked at us, sceptically, and asked: 'Can I see some ID, thanks?'

We all frowned and then stupidly, I began to laugh. 'You're joking, right?'

She shook her head. 'No, why would I be?'

I looked at Elli and my heart began to race. 'We're not eighteen,' I told her.

'Well then, you can't go through.'

The four of us looked around desperately and almost at the same time said, 'But we're supporting Dom!'

I added, 'We're on the poster – we just went and ate dinner.'

Her face was expressionless and her tone flat. 'I'm sorry, but we don't allow minors after eight.' I checked my phone. It was seven thirty.

Dom came to see what all the fuss was about; by this time I was almost yelling, and Elli and Chelsea were trying their best to calm me down. I could feel the tears welling. Dom said calmly, 'I'm sorry, Grace. I didn't realise it'd be a problem.'

I remember standing on the street, bawling my eyes out.

I remember telling Elli in between sobs, 'I'm so ... *tired.'*

I remember Dad pulling up in the car, and the look of frustration on his face as I relayed the story.

People arrived; friends who had travelled for hours to come and see us play. I felt ... guilty as I told them, 'Sorry, but we aren't allowed to do the gig.' I saw tears in Annie's eyes, and I remember thinking, *All I want to do is sing.*

Elli's dad arrived, and suggested we play anyway. 'I didn't ride my bike all this way for nothing, kids. Come on, you can have my helmet for money.' Elli was not keen. Chelsea and I begged her, told her it would be totally worth it.

'Okay,' she said. Heart racing, I hugged her and told her I loved her.

I remember skipping to the car and telling Dad and the look on his face, and the tone in his voice as he said, 'Don't be *fucking* ridiculous!' I wanted to cry again, and I wondered, Why doesn't he want to see us play?

I walked slowly back, head hung low. Elli held me by my shoulders and said, 'Grace, it's okay. We're going to do this.'

I remember standing in front of the little crowd, bike helmet and set list at my feet. I told them, 'Because we're little, we're not allowed to play inside. We're called Darling Street and this is Luke's song, "Emotionless Motion".'

I sighed and laughed and I remember having cold feet.

I remember the looks on everyone's faces. Especially Annie's. She was smiling and suddenly it all seemed worth it.

Dad stayed in the car.

We made $30 and everyone was proud

In the car on the way home, I hardly spoke. It was a bittersweet feeling, and even though he tried to joke about it all, even though he thought that it had been okay to not see me play my first gig – I couldn't be angry.

I could never *really* be angry.

Just ... disappointed.

The next little bit

I was feeling much better, particularly considering I'd finished year eleven. Dad was home, just in time for my departure. Annie and I had been planning a camping trip for weeks. We'd booked a site at the Goolwa Caravan Park and I was excited by the prospect of swimming, surfing and scouting.

Oh, and being totally free (for seven days, but still).

Noble Avenue

And totally free is exactly what we were.

We had quite the epic time – laughing and drinking and whingeing about the shit weather and swimming and driving and doing silly things (like putting our numbers under the windscreen wiper of a car with P plates) and taking hundreds of photos and walking and eating and listening to the same songs over and over and over and *over* and realising that maybe we should have just booked a cabin and telling stories and telling lies and telling each other that *yes you* should *buy that dress* and spending lots of money on really pointless things and straightening our hair and getting sunburnt and hugging and giggling and wondering and wandering and sighing and playing board games and drawing silly pictures and *forgetting.*

That was the main thing.

Epilogue

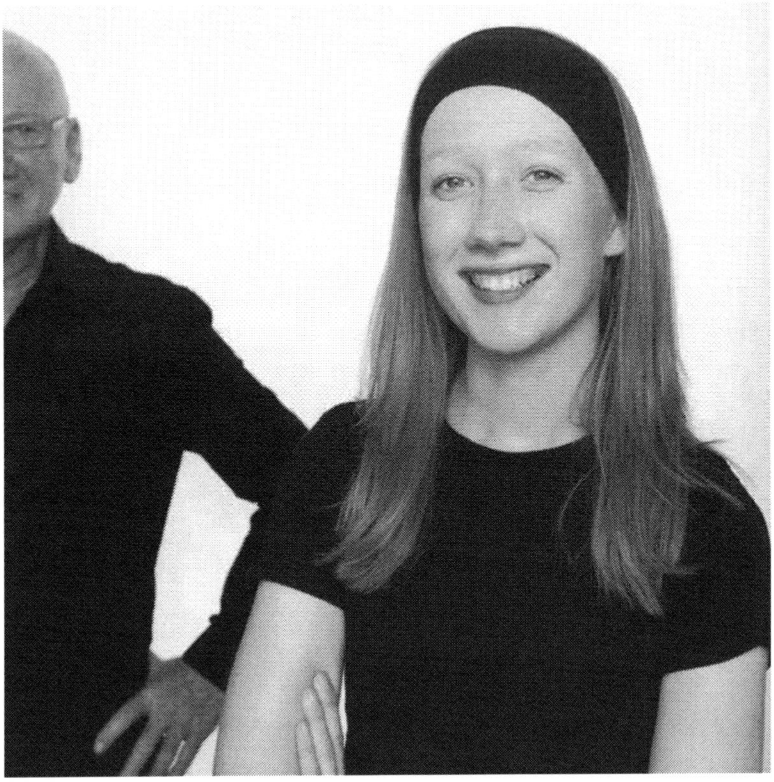

Once upon a time, when the birds chewed lime and the monkeys chewed tobacco – he was not okay.

He taught me how to be afraid, and how to be patient, and how to make the perfect cup of tea. He showed me how to be brave, how to get to North Wing, and the best way to position his pillows. (And also that it is okay to *not* feel brave, sometimes.)

He had radiation forty-five times, although it felt like a hundred. It was supposed to get rid of the lump (and make his neck a little bit red).

I cried because I hated hearing him say, *I don't know if I can do this anymore.*

He read me appointment times for chemotherapy. He sighed after each one. I bought Lean Cuisine for dinner and he let me stay at home by myself so I knew what a world without him would be like.

But I didn’t have to know – not for long.

Because he got better.

Geoff Goodfellow

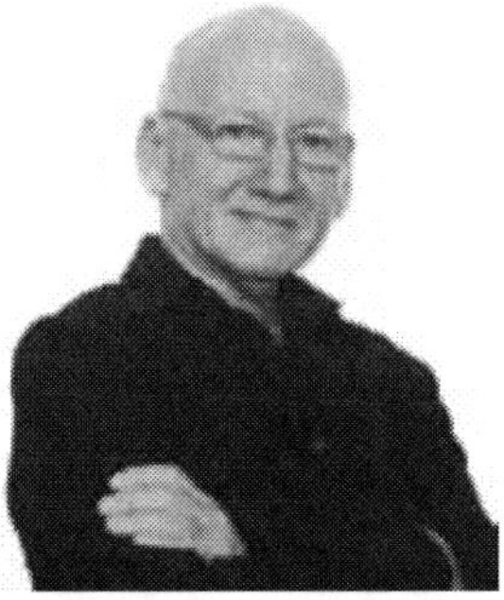

Geoff Goodfellow's writing career spans twenty-five years. His poetic observations of working-class Australian culture feature in his nine books, most of which have gone into multiple print runs. His *Poems for a Dead Father* was short-listed for the 2002 *Age* Book of the Year Award.

Geoff has performed nationally on building sites, in factories, jails, rehabs, schools, colleges, universities, and a wide variety of interesting and unusual places. He has travelled extensively on reading tours including to Cuba, USA, Canada, UK, Europe and China, appearing at literary festivals and often taking up positions as writer-in-residence at various institutions. His career has included bouts as writer-in-residence in a diverse range of places from York University in Toronto to Yatala Labour Prison in Adelaide.

On 1 February 2008, Geoff was diagnosed with cancer of the throat. *Waltzing with Jack Dancer: a slow dance with cancer* is a narrative of his survival.

poetforhire@picknowl.com.au
www.geoffgoodfellow.com

Grace Goodfellow

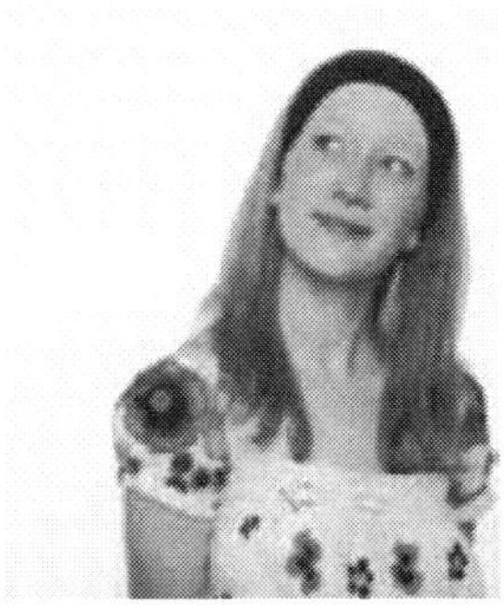

Grace Goodfellow, lover of lists, stories and stealing lines from conversations, began writing as soon as she was physically able. In 2008, she was awarded the overall prize for The Somerset National Novella Writing Competition.

She believes that family members and friends of those suffering with cancer suffer just as much pain.

This is partly why writing 'The C Word' was so important to her (and she needed a Christmas present for her dad).

Grace is studying Early Childhood Education at the University of South Australia, still sings in the band Darling Street and lives with her dad, Geoff, in a little suburb by the sea.

Randy Larcombe

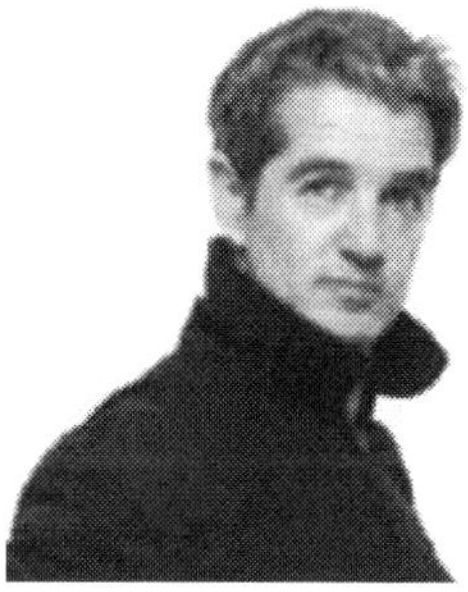

Randy Larcombe has worked as a professional editorial and commercial photographer since 1994. His love of photographic portraiture was rewarded early in his career with inclusion in *TIME, The Bulletin, Good Weekend Magazine, Weekend Australian Magazine* and *Australian Geographic.* For over a decade his work has featured in *Sunday Life, Wallpaper*, Forbes, Travel and Leisure, Women's Weekly, The Financial Times UK, Sumptuous* and *Adelaide* Magazine.*

Randy first met Geoff on a photoshoot for *Good Weekend* in 2001. On discovering they frequented the same coffee shop their acquaintance grew. When Geoff's cancer was diagnosed it seemed a logical path to document his journey.

His cover portrait of Geoff Goodfellow was shortlisted in the 2009 Moran Contemporary Photographic Prize. In 2009 Randy was voted by his peers to be among the Top 10 Commercial/Industrial Photographers in Australia.

Randy Larcombe is based in Adelaide and travels extensively throughout Australia for work and to pursue his personal photographic projects.

www.randylarcombe.com.au

Wakefield Press is an independent publishing and distribution company based in Adelaide, South Australia.
We love good stories and publish beautiful books.
To see our full range of titles, please visit our website at
www.wakefieldpress.com.au.

Back Cover Material

Geoff Goodfellow is one of those rare people who says what he thinks, usually with a few expletives added. When he learned he had cancer, he told the disease what he thought of it, and like a boxer, prepared himself for the fight ahead. Yet Geoff is also a sensitive man whose poems tap into the emotions unleashed by a close encounter with death. Randy Larcombe's photographs are a perfect match. They are brutally honest about the impact of cancer and the treatment of it, and at the same time they are deeply moving because they reveal the human frailty of this proud man.

Roy Eccleston

I have admired tough nut Geoff Goodfellow's work in both the building and poetry caper from a careful distance for years. No matter what he pulls out when he opens his tool box, whether it's an HB pencil and a blank sheet of paper, or a claw hammer and spirit level, you know they will be put to good use. Whenever Geoff starts banging away it is always worth a good hard look. Have a read of 'The Seventh Doctor', it's a cracker.

H.G. Nelson

Cancer is an experience that should be avoided. Those unlucky enough to be affected expect the best of care, for their cancer and for themselves, as people. These poems recount a journey through one man's experience of cancer and its care. I recommend it to all patients, families and friends of those who have similiar experiences. In particular I recommend it to all those who care for those with cancer – giving time, humility and a holistic approach is essential for the best of care.

Guy Rees MBBS FRCS FRACS

Grace Goodfellow's wise, funny, sad story about her father's journey with cancer will move you deeply, unless you are carved from ice. I recommend it highly.

Brigid Lowry

Books For ALL Kinds of Readers

At ReadHowYouWant we understand that one size does not fit all types of readers. Our innovative, patent pending technology allows us to design new formats to make reading easier and more enjoyable for you. This helps improve your speed of reading and your comprehension. Our EasyRead printed books have been optimized to improve word recognition, ease eye tracking by adjusting word and line spacing as well as minimizing hyphenation. Our EasyRead SuperLarge editions have been developed to make reading easier and more accessible for vision-impaired readers. We offer Braille and DAISY formats of our books and all popular E-Book formats.

Printed in Dunstable, United Kingdom

91342914R00087